MW00714081

T'ai Chi

Sue Mackie

Contemporary Books, Inc.
Chicago

Library of Congress Cataloging in Publication Data

Mackie, Sue.
  T'ai chi.

  Includes index.
  1. T'ai chi ch'uan.   I. Title.
GV505.M325   1983   796.8'155   83-14355
ISBN 0-8092-5479-4

To Franz

Designed by Jill Raphaeline

Copyright © 1981 by Sue Mackie
All rights reserved
Published by Contemporary Books, Inc.
180 North Michigan Avenue, Chicago, Illinois 60601
Manufactured in the United States of America
Library of Congress Catalog Card Number: 83-14355
International Standard Book Number: 0-8092-5479-4

Published simultaneously in Canada by Beaverbooks, Ltd.
195 Allstate Parkway, Valleywood Business Park
Markham, Ontario L3R 4T8 Canada

This edition published by arrangement
with David Ell Press Pty Ltd, Australia

Contents

Acknowledgements

The assistance of the Australia-China Council in the form of a grant for the completion and publication of this book is gratefully acknowledged.

I would like to thank the publishers of *Zenyang Lianxi Taijiquan*, Shanghai Renmin Chubanshe, for allowing me to translate and use the material on t'ai chi techniques from that book.

On a more personal note, I would like to express my gratitude and appreciation to my t'ai chi teacher, Liu Jian, for his grace and inspiration, and to Margaret Cook for her timely and valuable encouragement.

Foreword

T'ai chi is an art and a science, and is becoming increasingly widely known and practised in Australia and the West. It is the art of shadow-boxing which has fascinated many spectators, rhythmic and fluid, conveying a sense of inner tranquility. It is a science of control of physical and mental functions that improves the health and outlook of the performer. This introduction by Sue Mackie should help to popularise t'ai chi still further.

The basis of this book is a Chinese text *Zenyang Lianxi taijiquan* ('How to Practise T'ai Chi') published by the Shanghai Education Press. This book is widely used in China by people wanting to learn, develop and enjoy t'ai chi. The Chinese publishers have agreed to the translation of part of their text for publication in English, and have expressed their pleasure that the work will now become accessible to a wider audience.

During the past few months the Australia-China Council has encouraged dialogue between Australian and Chinese publishers, by exchanges of delegations between the publishers associations of both countries. Discussions have been held on several possible areas for co-operation. It is encouraging to see one practical fruit of these discussions appear so soon after the exchange of visits.

There are many books on t'ai chi already available, but this is the first to be translated directly from a contemporary text used in the People's Republic of China, so it has the original flavour of t'ai chi as it is practised for health and enjoyment by millions of people in China, not diluted or modified to overseas taste.

The Australia-China Council has been established by the Australian Government to improve understanding and friend-ship between Australia and China in all areas. T'ai chi is one such area where we are pleased to have been able to bring about a meeting of minds, by means of a grant to assist with this publication by David Ell Press.

Dr. Jocelyn Chey
Executive Director
Australia-China Council

PART 1
WHAT IS T'AI CHI CH'UAN?

1. A Windblown Willow

T'ai chi ch'üan exists, not in the form, but in the spirit.
T'ai chi ch'üan exists, not in the external, but in the
internal; it stresses consciousness, not form.

Can it be, then, that t'ai chi ch'üan is meditation, an activity of
the spirit which requires the body to be motionless?

T'ai chi ch'üan is the martial art of inner power, of the
hard residing in the soft, of toughness harmonising with
gentleness. In it, strength resides in grace. Relaxed grace is
the beginning: strength is transformed into grace, the sum
of grace becomes strength and strength reverts to grace.

Think of how water supports a vessel. Such is t'ai chi's springing
power: a physical attitude of seeming-to-be-relaxed-yet-not-
relaxed.

Its motion coils, entwines and spirals, taking shape as arcing,
bowing movements that flow liquidly into each other without
the slightest trace of effort or force. Each posture is born in the
instant of seeming-to-pause-yet-not-pausing of the previous
stance.

Yet it is not a dance.

Exercising, stretching and clearing the whole body at its deepest levels, it is a combination of martial arts, artistry, preventive medicine and meditation.

Opinions vary widely as to just how old t'ai chi ch'üan is. Tradition has it that it originated with a Taoist monk by the name of Chang San-feng, who may have lived anywhere between 600 AD and 1600 AD.

There are other versions of when and by whom t'ai chi was created, but so far none of them can be said to be indisputable. Current opinion in mainland China attributes the creation of t'ai chi chüan to Ch'i Chi-kuang (1528-1587), who drew together into a formal canon the various schools of martial arts or boxing forms popular during the Ming dynasty.

T'ai chi ch'üan is actually a combination of three ancient Chinese skills:

Ch'üan Shu—coordinated movements of hands, eyes, body and feet;
T'u Na Shu—deep breathing from the abdomen to empty out the old and take in the new; and
Tao Yin Shu—bowing, lifting, crouching and stretching of the limbs.

It is concerned essentially with four matters:

the cultivation of ch'i and the hoarding of power;
there is softness in the midst of hardness;
the internalising of the spirit;
consciousness is held in the tan t'ien.

There are many, many styles of t'ai chi and each of them has its own characteristics. These variant styles have developed over the years much as dialects of a language do, changing with distance and time to become unique to an area or a particular master.

Yet they all spring from a common source and they all adhere to the principles of change and yin-yang. In the yin-yang symbol, now quite familiar to Westerners, there is in the yin (dark) half of the symbol a dot of yang (light), and in the yang half a dot of yin.

The concepts of change and yin-yang polarity are seen throughout t'ai chi, as for instance with concrete and hollow, where there is continual change (transformation) between concrete and hollow, and there is always hollow in the midst of concrete and concrete in the midst of hollow.

Generally identified by the family names of the masters who originated them, there are five main variant styles: the Yang, the Ch'en, the Sun and two Wu styles (having the same sound, but written with two completely different Chinese characters).

The Yang style is slow and gentle, with an expansiveness and ease of movement both agile and stable. It is one of the large-stance styles. The simplified 24-posture cycle described in detail in Chapter 6 is a Yang style t'ai chi, as is the 88-posture cycle widely practised in mainland China at present. (A list of the 88 postures is given in the Appendix.)

A combination of fast and slow, hard and soft, is what distinguishes the Ch'en style. Although new stances, old stances, large and small intermingle, it also is regarded as a large-stance style.

Of the two Wu styles, one is a small-stance style and the other a medium-stance style. In the small-stance Wu style, movements are small, compact and quick, and leg movements nimble and brisk. Moderate-sized stances, gentleness and compactness are the characteristics of the other Wu style.

The Sun style is quite similar to the small-stance Wu style in that its movements are small and compact, with a lively gait and agile use of the body.

Since what mostly distinguishes one style from another is tempo and whether its stances or postures are large, small or medium, the basic principles and techniques of t'ai chi as they are described in Chapter 10 are universal. They are applicable to each and every style of t'ai chi, just as are yin-yang and change.

It is difficult—if not impossible—to describe t'ai chi ch'üan to someone who has not seen it. Because they are lineal and sequential, written instructions simply cannot convey the dynamism, the beauty and the flow of t'ai chi's graceful yet strong motion. And the sense of somewhat static posturing which photographs pluck from the movements of t'ai chi is quite alien to its intrinsic mobility.

The way to know what t'ai chi ch'üan is is to see it happening, to feel it and to do it yourself. To become a windblown willow.

2. Ch'i

An essential aspect of t'ai chi is to cultivate *ch'i* so that it flows throughout the body, clearing the body's channels of any blockages and restoring it to a harmonious and natural balance. This cultivation of *ch'i* requires a degree of concentration that renders inactive those parts of the brain associated with normal daily activity, thereby allowing them to rest and recuperate.

Ch'i, incidentally, should not be confused with *chi*. Despite their similarity in romanisation and in pronunciation (to the Western ear), these two words have completely different meanings and are written with two completely different Chinese characters. *Ch'i* (pronounced *chee*) means both breath and vital energy; *chi* (pronounced *jee*) as in t'ai chi ch'üan means the utmost point, or the ultimate.

A precise definition of *ch'i* cannot be given, simply because it is not certain what *ch'i* actually is. People who feel *ch'i* flowing through the body experience physical sensations such as tingling, heat, expansion or a feeling like that of insects or ants crawling over the skin. These sensations are similar to those experienced by patients receiving acupuncture treatment and are described by acupuncturists as *the desired sensation*.

According to Chinese medicine, *the blood is the mother of ch'i* and *when ch'i moves so does the blood, when ch'i is obstructed so is the blood.* The movement of *ch'i* throughout the body, therefore, seems to be closely related to that of the movement of blood.

Ch'i could be conducted either as bio-electric pulses or through the network of main and collateral channels which acupuncture presupposes to cover the entire body. It is considered by some Chinese to be excitation of the sensory nerves caused by the internal and external stimulation of the body during the movements of t'ai chi.

Ch'i, or *inner ch'i*, is thus activated by the stretching and contracting of muscles and by bio-chemical and bio-electric changes in the body. These muscular contractions and changes in the body stimulate the blood capillaries, which excite the surrounding sensory nerve fibres in such a way as to produce the sensations associated with the movement of *ch'i*—tingling, heat, etc.

Try this simple technique of *blood level movement:*

Stand with feet a little further apart than shoulder width. Raise both arms out from the sides of the body until they are straight out and level at shoulder height. Then, with the whole body relaxed, very slowly bend the body sideways over to the left then slowly back up and over to the right so that the arms move slowly up and down like a seesaw.

Keep seesawing very slowly until the point is reached where the arm that is then down alongside the body feels hot and distended and starts to redden, while the arm then above your head starts to go white. At this stage, slowly straighten up.

When the arms return to their original position, stretched out sideways from the shoulders, the arm that was white will feel a sensation like that of insects crawling over the skin, or a warm swelling: this is *ch'i* moving.

To feel *ch'i* moving in the legs, adopt a hollow stance (see photo 5, page 48), standing very firmly with your whole weight on one leg. With heavy shoulders and hanging elbows, the *ch'i* will be able to sink to the small of the back and the abdomen. By relaxing the small of the back and the hips, restraining the buttocks, holding the torso centred and upright with knees bent and the knee caps pulling very slightly inwards, *ch'i* will then be able to reach right down to the toes of the leg your weight is on. You should again experience in that back leg the sensations associated with the movement of *ch'i*.

Certain conditions are necessary to bring the body's internal channels to the state wherein *ch'i* is able to flow or to move through them: your attention must be focused exclusively on what you are doing; the muscles must be relaxed; movements must be made slowly and smoothly; and consciousness—not effort—must guide all movements.

It should be pointed out, however, that not everybody experiences the sensations associated with the movement of *ch'i* through the body. Some people feel *ch'i* fairly soon after they are introduced to t'ai chi; with others it takes a much longer time, and there are some who never experience it.

It must not, of course, be presumed that someone who feels the sensations associated with the flow of *ch'i* is in any way 'better at' t'ai chi than someone who does not. Whether or not these sensations are experienced has a great deal to do with individual differences in physical constitution.

It is not *ch'i* alone which allows t'ai chi to heal in so many ways, and the absence of any sensation of *ch'i* should not be taken as a sign that it is not in fact moving through the body's internal channels.

So if you don't feel *ch'i* moving when you are doing t'ai chi, don't try to force it. The benefit you derive from t'ai chi as a preventive and a therapeutic exercise depends on your guiding all movements with consciousness rather than with effort; it does not depend on whether *ch'i* can actually be felt moving through the body.

3. Mentally, Physically and Spiritually

Mentally ...

There is something almost magical about t'ai chi ch'üan. More than just a physical exercise, it is a complex series of postures involving the conscious participation of every part of the body in gentle spiralling, rounded and controlled movements. Flowing at a constant and slow tempo, these movements coordinate with either flow or counterflow abdominal breathing to create within you a wonderful balance and sense of calm.

The harmonising of movement and stillness in t'ai chi demands utter involvement in physical movement. It demands a focusing of attention, a concentration of consciousness and an absorption of spirit to the extent that those parts of the brain not associated with physical movement are temporarily put out to grass and allowed a well-deserved rest. A round of t'ai chi can refresh you so much that the inside of your head sometimes feels as though it has just been rinsed with pure, clean water.

One of the delights of t'ai chi is that it can never be perfected, in the sense that you have exhausted all that it has to offer. Of course it can be done mechanically and thoughtlessly once you are conversant with the rudimentary movements. But to do it as it should be done, you must devote your attention exclusively to what you are doing, no matter how well you know the movements. You must always be *there*.

Learning the movements and postures is just the very beginning of the practice of t'ai chi. Once you feel reasonably comfortable with the basic physical movements, you can then begin the delightful and absorbing task of shaping them so that: *internal and external harmonise; upper and lower move in accord; all is integrated; consciousness moves and the body goes along with it; breathing is natural; once in motion there is no place that does not move.* There is an utter fascination and joy to be found in gradually welding spirit, feeling, sight, hearing, sense of touch, etc. into an integrated whole with bodily movements.

If this sounds like hard work ... well, it is. But it is hard work of a different kind—self-induced hard work that results in positive relaxation for mind, body and spirit.

... Physically ...

T'ai chi is one of life's rarities: it is enjoyable, *and* it is good for you. It really is not just an illusion that you feel good when you do t'ai chi. Our bodies know instinctively what is good for them and what is not; they react favourably to the former, adversely to the latter. The answer, then, is to become aware of our bodies and listen to what they are telling us.

The human body is capable of very strenuous physical activity and, although it puts up with a great deal over long periods of time, if it is not used affectionately and effectively its capabilities wither away and many of its functions eventually atrophy. We human beings are extremely durable and hardy specimens, however, and it often takes many years before physical and mental damage reaches saturation point and becomes manifest as illness or disease.

> Excellent health; indifferent health; poor health
> Youth; middle age; old age
> Pregnancy
> Mental fatigue; sedentary work; depression; nervous
>   debility
> Pre-menstrual tension; period cramps; period pain;
>   interruption of the normal menstrual flow

Neuralgia
High blood pressure; low blood pressure; anaemia
Insomnia
Heart trouble
T.B.
Arthritis; rheumatism
Flat feet
Hard physical labour
Diabetes
Stomach and gastric disorders
Haemorrhoids
Seminal emission

A formidable list. Yet t'ai chi will benefit anyone in the grip of any of these conditions.

More frequently and more urgently than ever before, we are being warned that our bodies need exercise, exercise and more exercise. This is because in our urban Western society physical exercise is no longer an integral part of our everyday activities, but must be sought as an end in itself. How many of us have the time these days to exercise as part of our daily routines: to walk to the shops, to walk when we visit friends or go to the theatre, to walk to and from work, or to do hard physical labour?

We are basically creatures of habit; even people who lead what seem to be very full and active lives pursue the same line of work, the same sports and the same leisure activities week after month after year. Even if we are able to fit in a daily round of physical jerks or an hour at the gym, what happens is that the same few muscles and the same parts of our bodies are used daily or exercised regularly, while other muscles and other parts of the body are quite untouched by it all. Some of them, in fact, might reside in someone else's body for all the care and attention we give them.

Normally healthy people will derive great benefit from calisthenics, which are excellent for getting the blood moving and the lungs working. But what about other parts of the body. Do the joints, for instance, get proper massage and exercise when we do calisthenics, or are they just put under sudden stress and severe strain? And what about the mind, the spirit, the emotions. Do they get their fair share of exercise and variation, too, or are they expected to survive and flourish on an unvarying and unpalatable daily diet of work, home, things to be done, daily worries and shopping lists?

Chinese medicine works on the premise that physical well-being is related to the free flow of the body's internal systems: *if there's pain then there's a blockage; if there's a blockage then there's pain.* Spiralling and twisting, entwining and coiling backwards and forwards, the gentle, slow movements of t'ai chi stretch out the arteries, veins and blood vessels as well as the muscles, tendons and ligaments of the entire body.

Instead of making the heart beat faster, as it does when subjected to the stress of a good hard physical workout, the slow gyrations of t'ai chi cause the heart to beat more strongly than when the body is at rest and circulate the blood more evenly through the veins than does ordinary exercise.

Thus, although the heart is exercised, no stress is placed upon it. People with heart trouble may feel a little fatigued after a round of t'ai chi, but, so long as they listen to their bodies and only very gradually increase the amount of energy they put into the movements, a little fatigue is nothing to be concerned about. Should palpitations or some shortness of breath be experienced while doing t'ai chi, don't panic and give up altogether, just take a break for a while. Remember that each time you do t'ai chi your heart will get that little bit stronger.

T'ai chi is very much an exercise designed to bring the body back into its natural balance. It aims to clear blockages in the blood circulation, in the lymph system, and in the circulation of the body's vital energy or *ch'i.* So it is not surprising that people suffering from high blood pressure will benefit as much from doing t'ai chi as will those suffering from low blood pressure. Both groups will find their blood pressure gradually normalising after they have been practising t'ai chi for some time.

A word or two to people with high blood pressure. When doing t'ai chi, be especially conscious that your movements are relaxed and that your spirit is quite calm. Mistakes and imperfections in movements can be corrected in time and postures gradually perfected. Don't rush through the postures, nor allow slips and mistakes to perturb you.

Pay particular attention to achieving *hollow upper* and *concrete lower.* In specific terms this means that the upper part of the body—shoulders, chest, arms, small of the back and abdomen—should be relaxed and the lower part of the body—the legs—should become the focus of tension. By doing this you will stabilise the lower part of the body and forestall any tendency for the blood to rush to the head, which happens when the head is heavy and the legs are light.

By improving circulation of the blood and gently exercising and relaxing the muscles, t'ai chi offers relief to women who suffer from pre-menstrual tension and/or painful menstruation: *if there's pain then there's a blockage.*

Muscular cramps develop when the muscles don't get sufficient oxygen to enable them to contract smoothly. T'ai chi's gentle, unhurried movements and emphasis on breathing deeply and relaxing the muscles give direct relief by helping to untie cramps, reduce congestion in the pelvic region and alleviate that dragging feeling in the gut and lower abdomen. The exercise afforded by t'ai chi and combined with abdominal breathing promotes gentle massage of the internal organs which, over a period of time, tones up the muscles of the vagina and uterus.

Constipation contributes greatly to discomfort in the abdominal region at any time, but particularly is this so during menstruation and pregnancy. Gentle, relaxed t'ai chi movements help overcome constipation by restoring the body's internal organs to a condition of balance where they function in a normal and healthy way.

Menstruation and pregnancy are times when a little extra self-love doesn't go astray. If, for instance, you suffer very badly from cramps, then just be a little gentler with yourself when doing t'ai chi and pay particular attention to using consciousness —not effort—to relax your abdomen and to breathing deeply and slowly from the abdomen.

Pregnant women should do the same and simply avoid or modify postures where they stand on one leg, e.g. in *13* and *15 Planting the Foot,* or lower themselves down towards the ground, e.g. in *16* and *17 Low Free Standing,* especially in the later stages of pregnancy.

For about a month after giving birth it may be a good idea to take a break from t'ai chi and do special exercises recommended by your clinic or medical adviser. Doing t'ai chi out of doors is excellent exercise for you if you are breast feeding, as it helps rebuild your strength and increases the calcium and phosphate in your milk.

It is quite normal for the legs to ache somewhat when you start learning t'ai chi because the bent-legged, slow movements are unfamiliar and do put quite a strain on the legs. T'ai chi is dynamic: once movement has commenced, at no time is the body motionless or static. Often the greater part or all of the body's weight is supported by only one leg; transitions from one posture to the next are made very slowly; the knees are bent the whole time; and there should eventually be differentiation in the legs between concrete and hollow.

In spite of this, or perhaps because of it, sufferers from arthritis and rheumatism respond very well to the continued practice of t'ai chi.

If you have arthritis or rheumatism, it is wise to take a short walk or do a few gentle warm-up exercises before doing an actual cycle of t'ai chi. Gradually joints will become less painful and capable of greater and freer movement as improved blood supply to the muscles improves muscle tone and the nutritional condition of tissue surrounding the joints, so that harmful and painful excitation of nerve endings is lessened.

As the pain eases with time, however, be very careful that your movements remain relaxed and gentle so that you don't put an inordinate and premature strain on the legs. You should very gradually increase the scope of the joints' movements and progress by easy stages so that the joints don't become red or swollen. It is quite normal for muscles to ache a little after you do t'ai chi, and initially there may be some pain in the joints. But so long as you proceed *gradually*, the exercise afforded by t'ai chi can only improve an arthritic condition.

The best times, but by no means the only possible times, to practise t'ai chi are in the evening and in the early morning.

Whether a round of t'ai chi just before bed promotes or inhibits sleep seems to vary from individual to individual. Try it out for yourself and if you find a pre-bedtime round of t'ai chi wakes you up too much, then do it two to four hours before going to bed.

In the early morning the air is fresh and still and a round of t'ai chi gently stimulates the body, centres and calms the spirit and helps set you up for the day ahead.

... and Spiritually

The spirituality of t'ai chi ch'üan is in the doing of it. It is in the awareness thus gained of the flow of transformation or change as it is expressed in bodily movement.

The answer to the question, 'What is the philosophy of t'ai chi ch'üan?' must be, 'transformation'. Becoming aware of transformation in physical movement, we may extend this awareness and see that it applies in nature, in our lives, in the entire universe. We may finally be able to bend and not break under the weight of the snow, be able to go with the flow, become one with the One, knowing we ourselves are the Tao.

A background in Chinese Taoism (pronounced *dow*-ism) is not necessary to the practice of t'ai chi ch'üan but, by providing a proper context, such knowledge does allow both a greater understanding of many of the concepts of t'ai chi ch'üan and an insight into the unique Chinese genius.

Ultimately, involvement in the practice of t'ai chi ch'üan is involvement in the principles of Taoism, for the philosophical or spiritual source from which t'ai chi chüan springs is Taoism.

Tradition has it that Taoism originated with Lao-tzu, the Old one, who lived in the 6th century BC, about the same time as Confucius. Whether or not it was actually written by Lao-tzu, the *Tao Te Ching* (pronounced *Dow Der Jing*) has always been accepted as the original and basic text of Taoism. Mainly by means of witty anecdotes and parables, Chuang-tzu, who lived some two centuries after Lao-tzu, expounded Lao-tzu's thoughts and has come to be regarded as co-founder with Lao-tzu of philosophical Taoism.

Taoism very quickly became so much a part of Chinese thought and culture that when Buddhism reached China about the first or second century AD its teachings were adapted to make it more acceptable to the Chinese by blending it with Taoism; it is this Taoist-influenced Buddhism (Ch'an Buddhism) which forms the basis of Zen, or Japanese Zen Buddhism.

Gradually adapted by the people of China, the philosophical Taoism of Lao-tzu and Chuang-tzu became over the centuries a somewhat different Taoism—religious Taoism. Religious Taoism was concerned less with philosophical speculation than with alchemy and certain mystical and usually secret practices. The essence of these practices was to cultivate and preserve one's *ch'i* or vital energy by assiduous practice of breathing techniques in order to become one with the One, with the Tao. A lesser goal was simple longevity or immortality.

Breathing techniques were gradually broadened to include physical exercises and martial arts. In these martial arts it was not brute strength which overcame, but the appropriate and clever use of the forces of nature such as momentum and balance, echoing the words of Lao-tzu that the soft overcomes the hard, and the weak overcomes the strong.

In recent times, soldiers of the armies of the Taiping Rebellion in the mid-19th century were skilled in martial arts, and the famous Boxer Uprising of 1900 was led by a group of martial artists who believed their mystical arts could render them immune to bullets and swords. Associated with the Boxers, incidentally, were two groups of women martial artists, the Red Lanterns and the Blue Lanterns, these names referring to the coloured lanterns traditionally associated with Taoism.

This, very simply and very briefly, is the family tree of t'ai chi ch'üan.

Modified though they be from those of earlier times, the movements of present-day t'ai chi ch'üan still relate to the philosophy of Taoism.

The meaning of the words t'ai chi is 'extreme ultimate' or 'great absolute'; the meaning of the word ch'üan is 'fist'. In the beginning was *Wu Chi* (*without ultimate*), the void out of which *T'ai Chi*, *extreme ultimate*, came into being. T'ai Chi in turn generated *yin* and *yang*, and it is through transformation or interaction between *yin* and *yang* that all things in the universe are created. T'ai Chi has thus come to be represented by the *yin-yang* circle, symbol of polarity and balance.

The movements of t'ai chi ch'üan (*Extreme Ultimate Boxing*) are infused with both polarity and balance: concrete/hollow, open/closed, exhalation/inhalation, upper/lower, in front/behind, ascending/descending, tension/relaxation. Throughout the entire cycle it is required that there be a continual transformation back and forth between concrete and hollow, between open and closed, between advancing and retreating, etc.

At no point in t'ai chi ch'üan is there absolute concrete or absolute hollow, absolute advancing or absolute retreating, absolute tension or absolute relaxation. There should always be hollow in the midst of concrete and concrete in the midst of hollow and so forth.

Put another way, there should always be *yin* in the midst of *yang* and *yang* in the midst of *yin*, just as there is a small dot of *yin* (dark) in the *yang* (light) half of the *yin-yang* circle and a small dot of *yang* in the *yin* half of the circle.

For in Taoist terms *yang* cannot exist without *yin*, the two are simply opposite poles of the same continuum. The seed of one is in the other and to move from one to the other requires not a leap or a break, but a transformation or a transition. This same principle holds for tension and relaxation, for exhalation and inhalation, for concrete and hollow, for good and evil, for beauty and ugliness.

To a Taoist, death is not the end, nor is it the beginning: it is simply a transformation from one state to another state.
For your own pleasure I would recommend that you read some books on or about Taoism. Some suggestions are given below as an introduction to this vast and fascinating subject.

The *Tao Te Ching* has been translated many, many times. Some reliable and enjoyable translations are:

The Way of life according to Laotzu, translated by Witter Bynner. (Editions Poetry London 2. London, Lyrebird Press, 1972).

The Way and its power: the Tao Te Ching and its place in Chinese thought, translated by Arthur Waley. (London, Mandala Books, 1977).

Tao Te Ching, translated and with an introduction by D.C. Lau. (Penguin, 1972).

The writings of Chuang-tzu are available in various translations, e.g.

Chuang tzu: basic writings, translated by Burton Watson. (New York, Columbia UP, 1964).

Chuang Tsu. Inner Chapters. A new translation by Gia-fu Feng and Jane English. (London, Wildwood House, 1974).

Particularly relevant to students of t'ai chi is a full translation of the T'ai Chi Ch'üan Classic which has recently been published under the title *The Essence of t'ai chi ch'uan: the literary tradition*, by Benjamin Lo, Martin Inn, Robert Amacker, Susan Foe (Richmond, Calif., North Atlantic Books, 1979).

There are many books on Taoism available in most public libraries, but probably the most accessible and readable is that written by Alan Watts with the collaboration of Al Chung-liang Huang, *Tao: the watercourse way* (London, Jonathan Cape, 1976).

PART 2
LEARNING T'AI CHI CH'UAN

4. Abdominal Breathing

T'ai chi is a therapeutic, healing exercise and the techniques adopted in t'ai chi breathing derive from another Chinese healing art. The techniques are that of expulsion and admittance of *ch'i* (*t'u na shu*) and that of guiding the *ch'i* (*tao yin shu*). The other healing art which uses these techniques is healing by inner strength, a system of deep breathing exercises with quite simple postures in which stress is placed on regulating breathing. The postures of t'ai chi, however, are very complicated, and until you have become thoroughly familiar with the movements it will not be possible to amalgamate them with abdominal breathing. So don't worry about trying to coordinate breathing and movements until the whole cycle of postures has been learnt.

At the start just breathe naturally, taking care only that the *ch'i* sinks to the *tan t'ien*. To allow the *ch'i* to sink to the *tan t'ien*, hold your body erect with a compact abdomen and broad chest and consciously direct your breath so that you feel it slowly entering the area 7 cm (3″) below the navel. Don't try to press it down forcefully into the abdomen; allow your movements to be very easy. Allow your spirit to quieten, your *ch'i* to gather and your nerves to open out—let all this happen completely naturally without any forcing whatsoever.

There are two methods of abdominal breathing—flow and counter-flow—which are explained in this chapter. Do a few consecutive rounds of flow or counter-flow breathing as both a preliminary to a cycle of t'ai chi and when the cycle has been completed. Having become accustomed to breathing in this way, you will find it easier eventually to combine breathing with movements—once you have become conversant with the latter.

For people whose time is limited, or whose health is not up to doing t'ai chi postures, this breathing exercise is most beneficial when practised regularly morning and evening, up to twenty minutes at a time. Sick people can do it several times a day as their health permits.

Counter-flow Abdominal Breathing

1. Stand erect, feet together, toes pointing directly ahead. Step sideways with the left foot until the feet are the same distance apart as the shoulders, toes still pointing straight ahead, knees with a slight natural bend, spinal column sitting firm and vertical and the weight distributed evenly on both legs. Toes, soles of the feet and heels are all in contact with the ground, inner thighs open and rounded. Fingers are separated naturally, fingertips hanging down alongside the outside of the thighs and elbows slightly bent at a natural angle. There should be enough space between the upper arms and the body to fit a fist under the armpit.

The *pai hui* acupuncture point on the very top of the skull (in line with the tips of the ears) feels as though it is reaching delicately upwards: it is as though a cord were attached to it, suspending it from above. Then imagine there is a bowl of water on your head. Focus on some distant point straight ahead and quietly listen to what is behind you. The lower jaw is drawn in slightly, lips lightly closed, teeth lightly together and tongue relaxed with its tip curled up slightly towards the upper palate. Breathe through the nose.

The neck is relaxedly erect, shoulders slightly heavy and held as though there were a cord threaded across through the shoulder joints. Collarbones are secure and chest expanded, neither concave nor convex. Abdomen is compact, i.e. *ch'i* has sunk to the *tan t'ien*.

2. With the whole body relaxed, consciously calm your spirit and your breathing. Raise both hands very slightly till they are in front of the groin, palms pressing downwards a little, fingers separated naturally, fingertips pointing ahead, knuckles raised slightly. Consciousness is directed to the fingertips and the underside of the fingertips are above the toes.

At the same time, curve your shoulders slightly forward, creating a slight tenseness across the back muscles: this is the attitude of holding the chest and drawing the back. The vertebrae of the spinal column sit heavy and vertical, giving strength to the base of the spine and making the abdomen compact. The big vertebra at the top of the spine pulls slightly upwards and backwards in a somewhat inclined plane in direct proportion as the tailbone pulls down.

This is the basic stance for t'ai chi, wherein the spirit is pure and peaceful, upper and lower are on one cord; there is a delicate guiding up of the strength of the crown of the head (suspended crown of the head) and *ch'i* sinks to the *tan t'ien*; the chest is held and the back drawn, shoulders are heavy and elbows hang; the small of the back is caved in and the groin relaxed, knees bent with a rounded crotch.

3. Continuing from this seeming-to-pause-but-not-pausing posture, slowly inhale and raise both hands forward at arm's length out past the toes till they are at shoulder level. Elbows are slightly bent, with the tips of the elbows pointing downwards, so that the arms stretch out in front to form a shallow arc. Meanwhile, the lower abdomen below the navel is gradually pulled in.

4. Slowly begin to exhale, immediately letting the tips of the elbows descend until they are in front of the ribs, upper arms not touching the body, hands still level with the shoulders. While drawing the hands in towards the body, turn the palms in towards each other slightly until the backs of the hands are facing outwards, with the space between the thumb and index finger rounded, palms hollowed and the fingers pointing upwards at an oblique angle.

5. The hands (turned slightly inwards) slowly continue on down in front of the body until they come to rest in front of the groin. Exhalation should be smooth and even. Meanwhile, gradually push the lower abdomen out, i.e. *ch'i* sinks to the *tan t'ien*.

6. Let the fingertips drop back down, relax the whole body and resume the original stance as in **1.**

7. Repeat the whole movement (**1** to **6**) a second and a third time.

Flow Abdominal Breathing

Flow abdominal breathing differs only in that, as the hands are raised level with the shoulders, *ch'i* is consciously directed down into the lower abdomen, which is allowed to *expand* naturally; on exhalation, as the hands are lowered, the abdomen *retracts* naturally; i.e. the movement of the abdomen is the opposite of that in counter-flow abdominal breathing, but everything else is exactly the same.

The way you use your body and breathe, as described above, is fundamental to t'ai chi and should be maintained throughout the entire cycle.

A few other basic points which are relevant to abdominal breathing, but which should always be kept in mind when doing t'ai chi, are:

- The first and most important point is to calm and relax your nerves and collect your thoughts so as to quieten the entire body, internally and externally.
- Direct your movements consciously, making them flow together at a uniform pace and with relaxed—not rigid—strength.
- Breathing should gradually become deep, long, thorough, slow, even and calm. Breathing and movements should harmonise.
- Gaze straight ahead into the distance, focusing on the hands as they rise up into and descend down from the field of vision, then immediately gazing off into the distance again. Don't lower your head to look at your hands but retain the attitude of suspended crown of the head. In this way the eyeball and optical nerves are put to work and receive their share of exercise.
- If your chest begins to feel tight, if you become short of breath, or if you feel heavy-headed, you should reassess your state of relaxation by going back to the beginning and starting again. If an unfavourable reaction is again experienced, stop for the time being and try again later.

Peristalsis

After practising abdominal breathing for some time, it is possible that you will become aware of gurgling noises in your stomach and abdomen. Should this occur, it will be especially evident in changing from one stance to another, when the small of the back and the groin are relaxing and rotating. This completely natural biological phenomenon is described in the T'ai Chi Classic as 'relaxing the intestinal region, the vapours bubble up', and is brought about by consciously directing the breath and allowing the *ch'i* to sink to the *tan t'ien*. What is happening is that the gaseous vapours of the stomach and abdomen are churned up by the peristaltic action which the rotation of the small of the back and the rising and falling of the diaphragm stimulate. The viscera benefit greatly from this stimulation and in time the gurgling will lessen, until it finally disappears. It is nothing to worry about.

5. The Movements and Postures

Preparation

All you need to start learning t'ai chi is a flat, empty space about 4.25 m (14 ft) × 1.25 m (4 ft), comfortable clothing, flat shoes or bare feet and quietness in which to concentrate on what you are doing. You don't have to wear special clothes; but don't wear a tight belt or pants with a close-fitting waistband or tight legs, as these restrict both movement and breathing.

T'ai chi can be practised indoors or outdoors, depending on what space is available to you. It is, of course, preferable to do t'ai chi indoors when it's windy, cold or wet, but it is absolutely wonderful to do it in a grassy spot with trees around whenever you get an opportunity.

Generally, a 3 to 5 minute warm-up is enough for a cycle of t'ai chi. Start off by taking a short walk to stretch the lungs and start the blood moving. Then do a few simple exercises to relax the muscles and tendons and open out the joints, e.g. bend forward from the waist; do a few knee bends; swing, kick or stretch each leg out in front and behind; standing on one leg hug the other knee to the chest; with feet fairly wide apart press down with the hands on the upper thigh and the knee of each leg in turn;

make circles with the arms, with the hands, with the lower leg.

How strenuously you warm up depends entirely on your own state of health and fitness. Everyone knows his or her own limits and there is absolutely no need to exhaust yourself before you even begin to do t'ai chi. The nature of t'ai chi is gentleness and harmony; it is not designed to put the body under stress.

You can then do a few rounds of abdominal breathing. Practising one or two isolated postures such as *Cloud Hands, Grasping the Peacock's Tail* or *Stroking the Wild Horse's Mane* is also a good centring preparation.

When doing t'ai chi the heart should be calm, *ch'i* gathered and the spirit concentrated; so think also of spiritual preparation Before you begin, stand quietly with half-shut eyes or gaze off into the distance and focus your attention on being still. Or, standing in the preparatory stance, relax all the joints of the body, one by one, from head to toe, until the whole body feels relaxed, the spirit is internalised, the heart is calm and *ch'i* is gathered.

Legs

When you start learning t'ai chi your legs will ache. This is because you will be moving them in an unaccustomed manner, keeping them bent as weight is shifted slowly from one leg to the other, and quite often supporting all or the greater part of the weight of the body on one bent leg.

But aching muscles in the initial stages are quite normal and the ache will disappear in time as your body becomes familiar with the movements, your heart becomes stronger, blood circulation improves and lung capacity increases. Muscular aches will be lessened if you don't over-exert yourself at the outset. Taking a short walk straight after doing t'ai chi sometimes helps sore leg muscles, too.

The slower the t'ai chi cycle is performed, the greater is the burden borne by the legs. So until you have mastered the movements and your muscles and joints have become stronger and more flexible, it is essential that the degree to which your legs are bent be increased only very gradually.

The height and tempo at which you do t'ai chi dictates the amount of effort expended: standing fairly erect and moving quickly demands far less effort than does sinking closer to the ground and moving slowly. The amount of effort expended should be only gradually increased over time. When doing a complete cycle, the height to which you lower the torso at the beginning should be maintained throughout. If it is altered halfway through, the rhythm of the whole cycle will be disrupted.

To begin with, bend your knees (keeping the torso erect and not leaning forward) so that your thighs are at an angle of no more than 40° from the perpendicular. This is a high stance. A medium stance is with the thighs angled at 65° from the perpendicular, and the lowest stance is with the thighs angled at 90° from the perpendicular.

With time and practice, as your muscles relax and strengthen, you will gradually be able to bend your knees more and more. As your stance gradually becomes lower, so all the joints in the lower body will bend more acutely and your muscles and tendons will pull and stretch to a greater degree.

Once you have begun to move in t'ai chi, the weight of the body is continually being transferred from one leg to the other so that at no time, other than in the *Rising* and *Gathering In* postures, is the weight of the body supported equally by both legs.

The Steps

There are eight basic steps in t'ai chi:
1. the horse stance
2. the T-step
3. the heel stance
4. the bow step
5. the hollow stance
6. the grinding step
7. the attacking step
8. the one-legged stance.

They occur in the following movements or postures of the 24-posture cycle:
1. *Crossed Hands* **(photo 150)**
2. moving from *Rising* into *Stroking the Wild Horse's Mane* **(photo 2)**
3. the half step forward into *Crane's Wings* **(photo 15)**
4. *Stroking the Wild Horse's Mane* **(photo 4)**
5. moving from *Stroking the Wild Horse's Mane—Left* into *Stroking the Wild Horse's Mane—Right* **(photo 5)**
6. moving from *Stroking the Wild Horse's Mane—Left* into

Stroking the Wild Horse's Mane—Right **(photo 6)**
7. *Low Free Standing—Left* **(photo 115)**
8. *Low Free Standing—Left* **(photo 117)**.

Bow Step

Of these eight stances or steps, only the bow step will be explained in detail here, since it occurs the most frequently and is the step which students find the most difficult to master.

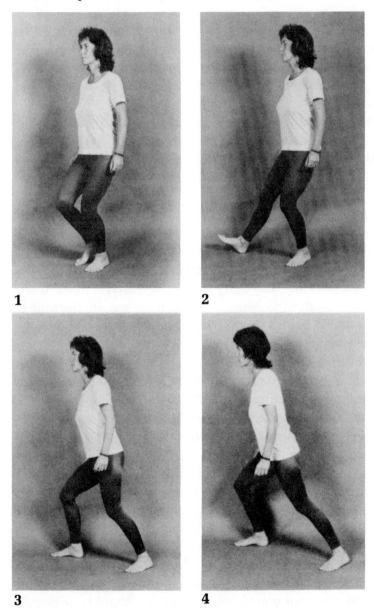

1

2

3

4

The description given here is of a right bow step. A left bow step is a mirror image of this, i.e. for left read right and for right read left.

Starting from the T-step **(photo 1)** with bent left leg and weight wholly on the left leg, the right knee lifts up a little, and the right foot slowly reaches out forward and very slightly to the right until the heel touches the ground.

At this point the buttocks are still directly above the left heel and the weight is still supported entirely by the bent left leg **(photo 2)**.

Then, as the sole of the right foot treads firmly down on to ground with toes pointing straight ahead **(photo 3)**, approximately 80 per cent of the body's weight gradually shifts forward on to the right leg, the right knee bends and the right leg bows, but only so far forward that the kneecap does not protrude beyond the toes.

The left foot remains wholly on the ground and presses firmly downwards, the left leg having a very slight bend in it. Its toes are still pointing forward but are angled a little out to the left **(photo 4)**.

Be careful to keep the hips level as your weight moves forward and do not confuse the thrusting up or out of the hip of the front leg with shifting your body weight from the back leg to the front leg. Nor is pushing the top of the body (head and shoulders) forward the same as shifting body weight foward on to the front legs. Shoulders and hips should slide forward in harmony, staying the same distance apart from each other, both horizontally and vertically.

As the right foot reaches out forward it also steps 10-30 cm to the right, as if stepping over a centre line. When the bow step is completed the heels are thus at a distance sideways from each other of 10-30 cm, and not on a straight line.

This serves two purposes. One is that it gives greater stability to the stance than if the feet were directly in line with each other. The other is that separating the feet makes it possible to bring the left hip around to the front as your weight shifts forward, so that in the completed bow step the abdomen is facing straight forward in the same direction as the toes and knee of the right leg.

In the early stages, the rear foot of a bow step can remain at an angle of up to 90° out from straight ahead, but with practice and as you learn to open out your hips, this angle should be lessened

until the toes of the rear foot point out at an angle of between 45°
and 60° from straight ahead.

Tempo

It has been said that a cycle of Wu or Yang style t'ai chi, such as
the 88-posture Yang style listed in the Appendix cannot be
executed under 50 minutes. Others say such a cycle should take
between 10 and 25 minutes.

The 24-posture cycle described in this book can take anywhere between 4 and 9 minutes to perform. A Ch'en style cycle
would normally take 5 to 8 minutes to execute, and between 6
and 15 minutes is usual for the Wu or the Sun styles.

As you can see, there is no absolute as to tempo: the right
tempo is one which is appropriate to an individual's constitution
and skill. However, if you do the movements of t'ai chi too
quickly they become blurred, frivolous and light; if you move
too slowly, on the other hand, it is difficult to keep the body in
motion, *ch'i* and gestures become too loose and the whole body
appears inert.

There is, though, some guidance to be had. With a quiet heart,
ch'i gathered and the body easy and relaxed, tempo should be
such that the tendons, bones and joints are gently stimulated
and *ch'i* can be felt flowing freely through the pulses.

How to Learn T'ai Chi

There are certain difficulties everybody experiences when they
start learning t'ai chi. It is best to be aware of these from the
outset so that they don't grow out of proportion and assume
undue importance.

The first and most obvious difficulty is trying to do everything
at once. T'ai chi may sound easy and it may look easy, but the
first few times you attempt it you'll wonder why you hadn't
noticed before how many limbs you have and why none of them
is able or willing to do what you want it to do. This will pass, so
don't let it worry you unduly.

Of course, everything *must* be done simultaneously; however,
in the initial stages it could help to break the movements down
into their component parts, learn those, and then reassemble
them as soon as you can into an integrated, flowing whole.

Grasping the Peacock's Tail—Left, for example, can be broken down into four parts, three of which coincide with the shifting backwards and forward of the body's weight:

the springing forward motion of the right hand **(photo 47, page 68)**;

the stroking motion down and to the side of both hands as weight shifts on to the back leg **(photo 48, p. 68)**;

the crowding forward motion of both hands as weight shifts on to the front leg **(photo 51, p. 69)**;

the pressing down motion of both hands as weight shifts on to the back leg **(photo 53, p. 70)**.

Most movements can also be broken down into what the arms and the upper part of the body are doing, and what the legs are doing.

A quite effective and comforting way of learning movements is to concentrate first of all on the steps, on what the legs are supposed to be doing. Put your hands on your hips (this is good practice for checking that the hips stay level, too) and quietly go through the motions of just the feet and the legs. This will usually involve turning the torso as you move, but, for the moment, you won't have to worry about the hands and arms.

Then, as soon as you feel you understand the leg movements, add in the movements for the upper part of the body.

It is less easy to isolate and practise hand movements, but it can be done in some postures. With *Cloud Hands*, for instance, the hand and arm postures only can be learnt first and then the legs added in; it sometimes helps with *Cloud Hands*, incidentally, to get one hand moving in the proper direction and then add the other hand in while you're learning this hand and arm action.

A second difficulty is keeping the legs bent and relaxed. There is usually a tendency for beginners to straighten each leg as the weight of the body falls on to that leg. The only advice that can be given is: always keep your legs bent. Try imagining you are in a room the ceiling of which just touches your head as you stand with bent legs. If you keep this image in your mind it may help you keep your head at the one height as you move from posture to posture and stop you bobbing up and down.

The Movements and Postures

In the description of the 24-posture t'ai chi cycle which follows, the principle enunciated by Mark Twain—*You can't do every-*

thing at once, but you can do something at once—has been adopted.

Bodily movements which are absolutely essential to completing a posture are printed in **bold type.** These basic actions of the arms and legs form the skeleton of each movement and posture and should be the first part of every movement attempted.

The instructions in ordinary type are those which should be incorporated once the basic movements have been mastered.

The instructions printed in brackets are not just niceties of style and form; they are an integral part of the movements. They can, however, be incorporated gradually as your skill and familiarity with the movements increases.

It is probably best to go through the whole cycle posture by posture, learning all the basic bodily movements so that you learn the whole cycle first in a correct, albeit approximate, fashion. Once the basic movements have been learned right through, then gradually incorporate the finer details, either while you are doing a complete cycle or by working on individual postures.

Remember, you cannot get everything right at once, so just relax and enjoy taking it step by step.

6. Simplified 24-Posture T'ai Chi

This Simplified T'ai Chi Cycle is based on the principle of working from the simple to the complex, from the easy to the difficult. It has been adapted and rearranged from various t'ai chi cycles from which superfluous repetitive movements have been removed in order to bring out the essential structure and technique of the original cycles and make it easier for the average person to learn.

There are eight Sections made up of 24 postures. The complete cycle may be practised, isolated postures selected as desired or separate sections performed as units in themselves.

Section 1
    1. Rising
    2. Stroking the Wild Horse's Mane—Left & Right
    3. Crane's Wings

Section 2
    4. Brushing the Knee Twist—Left & Right
    5. Strumming the Lute
    6. Reverse Unfolding the Arms—Left & Right

Section 3

7. Grasping the Peacock's Tail—Left
8. Grasping the Peacock's Tail—Right

Section 4

9. Single Whip
10. Cloud Hands
11. Single Whip

Section 5

12. Testing the Horse
13. Planting the Foot—Right
14. Twin Peaks Piercing the Ears
15. Revolving Planting the Foot—Left

Section 6

16. Low Free Standing—Left
17. Low Free Standing—Right

Section 7

18. Piercing the Shuttle
19. Needle Pointing to the Bottom of the Sea
20. Ducking through Arms

Section 8

21. Revolving Block Punch
22. As Though Sealing Up
23. Crossed Hands
24. Gathering In

In the description that follows, the words 'at the same time' mean that, regardless of whether certain parts of the body are mentioned before or after others, all bodily movements in each posture should be made at one and the same time. They must be made simultaneously, not one after the other.

If you do not have a teacher, however, it is helpful and encouraging when starting to learn t'ai chi to tackle the movements part by part. To make it easier, the following hints are given: the instructions in **bold type** are essential for attaining postures and for moving from one posture to the next; the instructions in ordinary type will put some flesh on the basic movements; and the instructions in brackets will clothe the movements and postures.

Follow these hints by all means, but always remember that this method is only a tool to help you reach the stage where all parts of the body move simultaneously and as a unified whole; once movement commences the cycle flows smoothly through to the final posture.

The direction of the movements is in relation to the practitioner's body: regardless of the rotation involved in the movements, in front of one's body is always forward, behind one's body is always backwards, to the left is left and to the right is right.

There are a few postures involving movements at rather oblique angles and for convenience it is assumed that the practitioner faces south at the commencement of the cycle so that in those cases where a more precise direction is necessary it can be given according to the points of the compass.

The photographs in the following description give a student's-eye view of the movements since when learning t'ai chi the student generally stands behind the instructor and attempts to duplicate the instructor's movements. By placing the reader in just that position, directly behind the instructor, there have arisen a few instances where the movements of the hands cannot be seen clearly; in these cases the student's-eye view has been supplemented by photographs showing the front or reverse view of those movements.

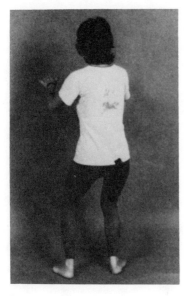

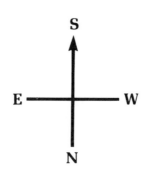

1

Section 1

Stand naturally erect, feet together, arms hanging easily by your sides so that the hands are at the outside of the thighs.
   Gaze straight ahead.

1. Rising

1. Step to the left with the left foot so that the feet are shoulder width apart, toes pointing straight forward. (Neck should be straight, chin pulled in slightly, chest not thrust out nor stomach pulled in.) Concentrated mind.

2. Both hands slowly lift forward at arm's length until they are shoulder high, shoulder width apart, palms facing down.

3. With torso remaining erect and weight distributed equally on both legs, **both legs bend at the knees (photo 1) into a slight crouch** (horse stance). (The small of the back should be relaxed, buttocks neither protruding nor tucked in.)

At the same time hands lightly press down and elbows drop down, bringing the hands in closer to the chest (**photo 1**). (Shoulders should be heavy, elbows dropping easily, fingers slightly bent.) Lowering of the body and of the arms takes place as a single movement.

Gaze straight ahead.

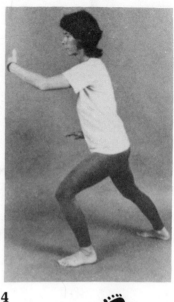

4

**2.
Stroking the
Wild Horse's
Mane—Left**

1. Torso turns very slightly to the right, **weight transfers on to the right leg and the left leg is brought in to the right instep** with the toes touching the ground (T-step) **(photo 2)**.
At the same time the right hand, palm down, **pulls up and in towards the chest, the left hand** (describes an arc down and across the front of the body) until it **is palm up beneath the right hand,** the two hands poised as if holding a balloon **(photo 2)**. (Gaze on right hand.)

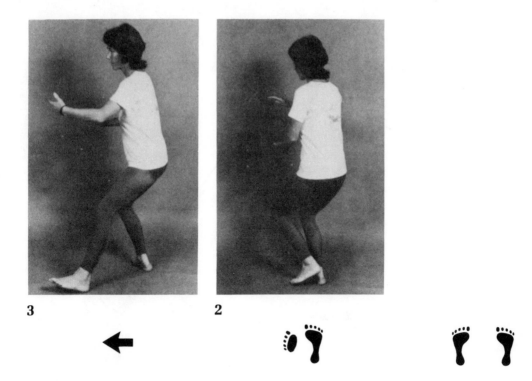

3   2

2. Torso turns a little to the left, **left foot steps out to the left, the right foot remains flat on the ground (photo 3)** as the right leg slowly straightens and about 80% of the **weight is slowly transferred on to the left leg** (left bow step) **(photo 4)**.

As the torso continues turning to the left, **the hands slowly separate** as they follow the body around, **the left hand being raised and the right lowered (photo 3)** until the left hand (palm facing up at an oblique angle) is at eye level and the right hand (palm facing down, fingers pointing forward) has fallen to level with the right groin **(photo 4)**. Both elbows are slightly bent. (Gaze on left hand.)

Direction: in this completed posture you will be facing left (or east) in relation to the Rising posture (south).

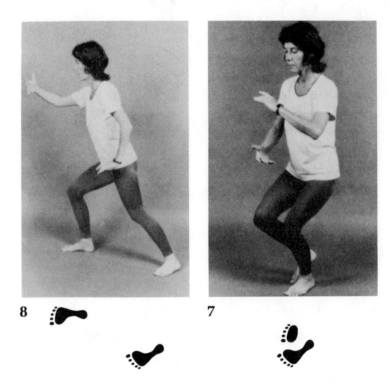

8   7

**2.
Stroking the
Wild Horse's
Mane—Right**

3. Torso slowly sits back, **weight transfers back on to the right leg and the left toes lift up and hook slightly out** 45°-60° (hollow stance) **(photo 5)**. **Then the whole left foot slowly treads right down,** left leg slowly bowing forward, body turns to the left and **weight transfers once more on to the left leg (photo 6) as the right foot is brought in towards the left instep** (grinding step). Then the toes touch the ground at the left instep **(photo 7)**.

At the same time the left hand turns in palm down and the **left arm pulls in towards the chest, while the right hand travels** (across in an arc) **to the left (photo 6)** until it is **palm up beneath the left hand,** the two hands poised as if they were holding a balloon **(photo 7)**.

(Gaze on left hand.)

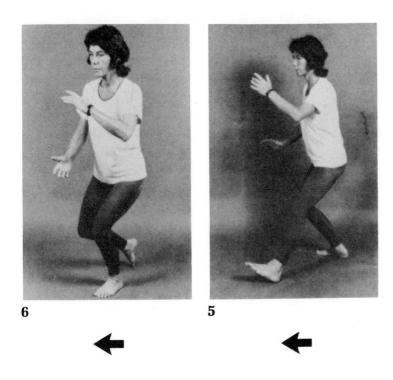

6   5

4. This movement is a mirror image of **Stroking the Wild Horse's Mane—Left (2):**
Right leg steps out forward to the right, the left foot remains flat on the ground and the left leg extends naturally as about 80% of the **weight is slowly transferred on to the right leg** (right bow step) **(photo 8)**.
At the same time torso turns to the right, **the hands slowly separate** as they follow the body around, **the right hand being raised and the left lowered** until the right hand (palm up at an oblique angle) is at eye level and the left (palm down, fingers pointing forward) has fallen level with the left groin **(photo 8)**. Both elbows are slightly bent.
(Gaze on right hand.)
Direction: in this posture you will again be facing east.

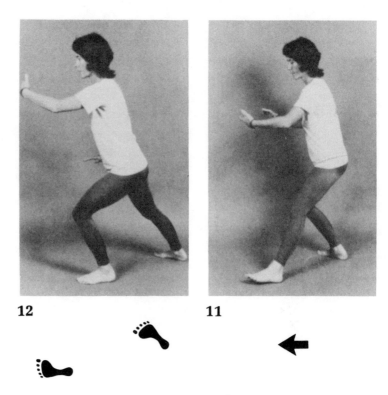

12   **11**

**2.
Stroking the
Wild Horse's
Mane—Left**

5. This movement is a mirror image of **Stroking the Wild Horse's Mane—Right (3)**:
Torso slowly sits back, **weight transfers back on to the left leg, right toes lift up and hook slightly out** 45°-60° **(photo 9), then the whole right foot slowly treads right down,** the right leg slowly bowing forward. Body turns to the right and **weight transfers once more on to the right leg. The left foot is immediately brought in towards the right instep** then the toes touch the ground at the right instep **(photo 10).**
At the same time the right hand turns in palm down and **the right arm pulls in towards the chest while the left hand travels** (across in an arc) to the right until it is **palm up beneath the right hand,** the two hands poised as if holding a balloon **(photo 10).**
(Gaze on right hand.)
6. This movement is exactly the same as **Stroking the Wild Horse's Mane—Left (2)**:
The left leg steps out forward to the left, the right foot remains flat on the ground (photo 11) and the right leg extends naturally as about 80% of the **weight is slowly transferred on to the left leg** (left bow step) **(photo 12).**

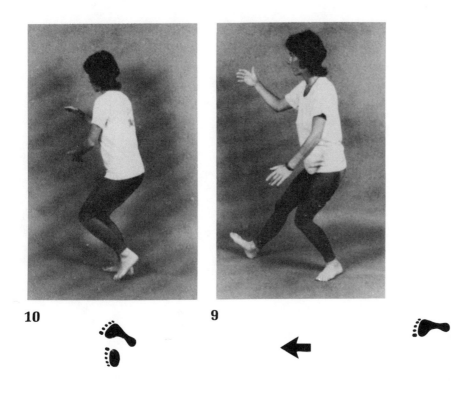

10   **9**

At the same time torso turns to the left, **the hands slowly separate** as they follow the body around, **the left hand being raised and the right lowered (photo 11)** until the left hand (palm up at an oblique angle) is at eye level and the right (palm down, fingers pointing forward) has fallen level with the right groin **(photo 12)**. Both elbows are slightly bent.
(Gaze on left hand.)
Direction: east

(Torso should be firm, chest broad and relaxed. Arms retain an arc shape as they separate. The small of the back is the fulcrum as the body turns. Arms and legs move as one.) With the bow step, **the heel of the forward leg touches the ground first;** the kneecap should not protrude beyond the toes and the toes should point straight ahead (east); the back leg is straight but not rigid; the back foot is at an angle of 45°-60° from the front (this angle can be obtained by pushing the heel of the back foot out a little). (With this bow step the heels should be 10-30 cm apart sideways, as if they were separated by a line running between them.)

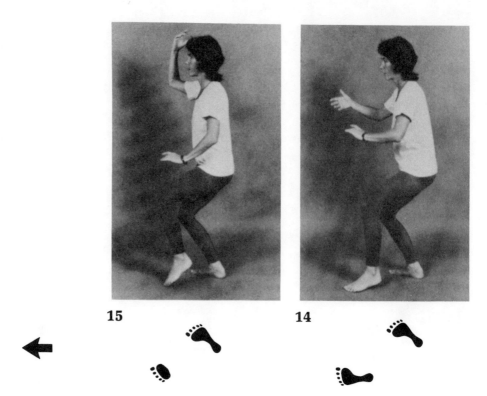

15   14

3.
Crane's Wings
(Torso turns slightly to the left) and **weight transfers wholly on to the front (left) foot. The right foot takes a half step forward (photo 13),** torso sits back as **the body's entire weight goes back again on to the bent right leg** (then torso turns slightly to the right) **(photo 14). The left foot then moves forward a little so that the toes are barely touching the ground** (left heel stance) (and torso turns back to the left a little) so that the body is finally facing straight ahead (east) **(photo 15).**

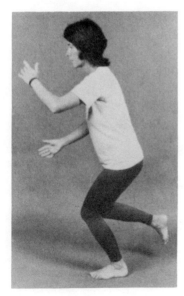

13

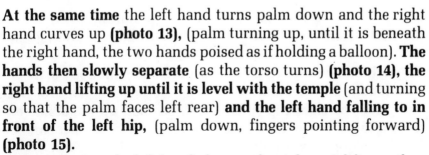

At the same time the left hand turns palm down and the right hand curves up **(photo 13),** (palm turning up, until it is beneath the right hand, the two hands poised as if holding a balloon). **The hands then slowly separate** (as the torso turns) **(photo 14), the right hand lifting up until it is level with the temple** (and turning so that the palm faces left rear) **and the left hand falling to in front of the left hip,** (palm down, fingers pointing forward) **(photo 15).**

(Gaze is first on the left hand, then on the right as it lifts up, then straight ahead.)

Direction: east

Chest should not be stuck out in this posture, arms always retain an arc shape and the left knee should be bent. (The movement of shifting the weight backwards takes place as the right hand lifts and the left falls.)

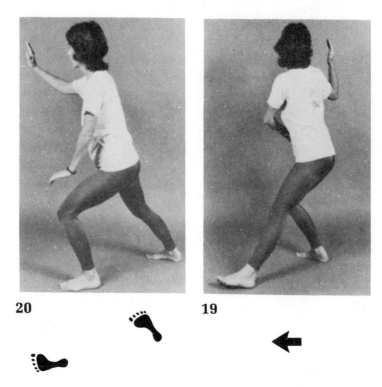

20   19

Section 2

**4.
Brushing
the Knee
Twist—Left**

1. (Torso first turns slightly to the left) **(photo 16),** (then back to the right) **(photo 17).** The left foot moves back in to touch the ground at the right instep **(photo 18).**
The right hand drops down across the front of the body to the left ribs (photo 16) then turns palm up (to describe an arc) **back alongside the right hip (photo 17) and then up to outside and behind the right shoulder (photo 18),** with the elbow bent and the hand pushing forward at ear level (palm obliquely up).
At the same time as the torso and the right hand are moving, **the left hand pulls back (photo 16) and up to shoulder level at the left (photo 17) then** (describes an arc) **across the front of the body to the right breast (photo 18)** (palm obliquely down).
(Gaze on right hand.)

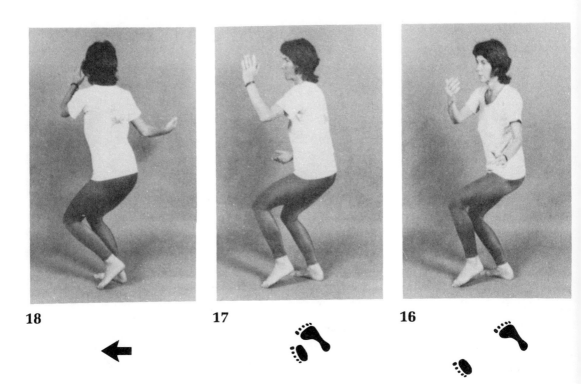

18   17   16

2. Torso turns to the left and **the left foot steps out forward and to the left (photo 19) to make a left bow step (photo 20).**
At the same time the right hand curves past the ear **(photo 19)** and **pushes forward level with the tip of the nose (photo 20),** **while the left hand drops down to the left across the body (photo 19)** (and brushes back from in front of the left knee) to come to rest alongside the left groin (fingers pointing forward) **(photo 20).** (Gaze on fingers of right hand.)
Direction: east

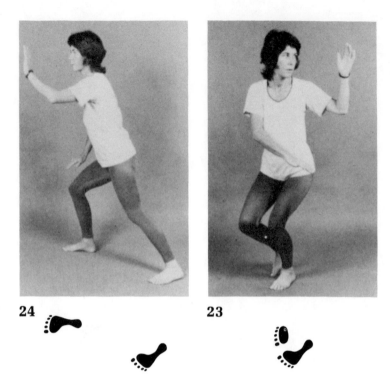

24   23

**4.
Brushing
the Knee
Twist—Right**

3. The right leg slowly bends at the knee, torso sits back and **weight transfers back on to the right leg. The left toes lift up and hook slightly out** (45°-60°) **(photo 21), then the whole foot slowly treads right down,** the left leg slowly bowing forward as the body turns left **and weight transfers once more on to the left leg (photo 22). The right foot is immediately brought in to the left instep,** toes touching the ground **(photo 23).**
At the same time the left hand turns palm up, (thumb leading it over **(photo 21),** and describes an arc) **back alongside the left hip (photo 22) and then up to outside and behind the left shoulder,** with the elbow bent and hand pushing forward at ear level (palm obliquely up). **The right hand travels** with the body, (describing a shallow arc up and then down) **to the left to in front of the left shoulder,** (palm obliquely down) **(photo 23).**
(Gaze on left hand.)

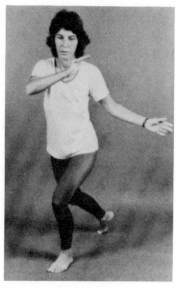

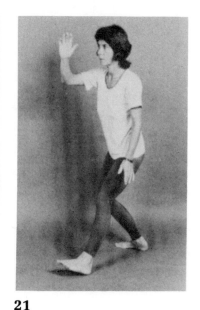

22   21

4. Torso turns to the right and **the right foot steps out forward
and to the right to make a right bow step (photo 24).**
At the same time the left hand curves past the ear and **pushes
forward level with the tip of the nose, while the right hand drops
down to the right across the body** (and brushes back from in
front of the right knee) to come to rest alongside the right groin
(fingers pointing forward) **(photo 24).**
(Gaze on fingers of left hand.)
Direction: east

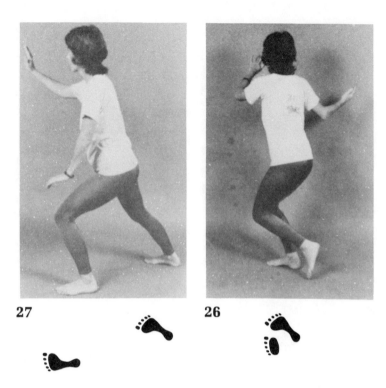

27   26

**4.
Brushing
the Knee
Twist—Left**

5. The left leg slowly bends at the knee, torso sits back and **weight transfers back on to the left leg. The right toes lift up and hook slightly out** (45°-60°) **(photo 25), then the whole foot slowly treads right down,** the right leg slowly bowing forward as the body turns right **and weight transfers once more on to the right leg. The left foot is immediately brought in to the right instep,** toes touching the ground **(photo 26).**

At the same time the right hand turns palm up, (thumb leading it over **(photo 25)**, and describes an arc) **back alongside the right hip and then up to outside and behind the right shoulder,** with the elbow bent and hand pushing forward at ear level, (palm obliquely up) **(photo 26). The left hand travels** with the body **(photo 25)**, (describing a shallow arc up and then down) **to the right to in front of the right shoulder,** (palm obliquely down) **(photo 26).**

(Gaze on right hand.)

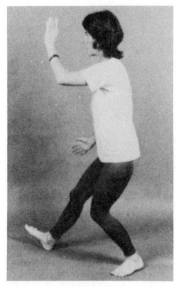

25

6. This movement is exactly the same as **Brushing the Knee Twist—Left (2):**
Torso turns to the left and **the left foot steps out forward and to the left to make a left bow step (photo 27).**
At the same time the right hand curves past the ear and **pushes forward level with the tip of the nose, while the left hand drops down to the left across the body** (and brushes back from in front of the left knee) to come to rest alongside the left groin, (fingers pointing forward) **(photo 27).**
(Gaze on fingers of right hand.)
Direction: east

When the leading hand pushes out forward, the body should neither bend forward nor lean backwards (and the small of the back and the groin should be relaxed).

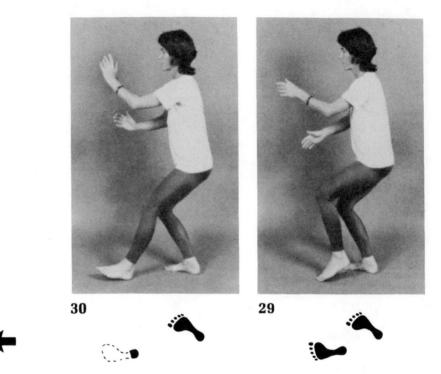

30   29

5.
Strumming
the Lute

Weight transfers wholly on to the front (left) foot. The right heel advances a half step (photo 28), torso sits back **and weight transfers back on to the right leg (photo 29).** (Torso turns to face half right) and **the left foot lifts** up a little to **move forward** to a left hollow step, **heel resting lightly on the ground, toes raised** and knee slightly bent **(photo 30).**
At the same time the left hand comes up at the left (photo 28) until it is level with the tip of the nose, (palm facing right) and elbow slightly bent **(photo 30). The right hand comes back in (photo 28) to rest alongside the inside of the left elbow,** (palm facing left) **(photo 30).**
(Gaze on index finger of left hand.)
Direction: east

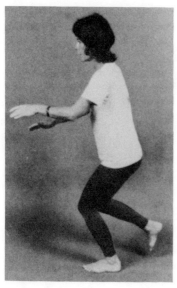

28

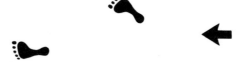

(Body should feel stable, shoulders heavy, elbows hanging and chest relaxed and full.) The left hand does not come up in a straight line, but has in its travel a hint of arcing up then forward. **When the right heel advances, it is the sole of the foot which makes contact with the ground first,** then the whole foot treads down. (The three actions of shifting the weight back, lifting the left hand and bringing the right hand in all take place at one and the same time.)

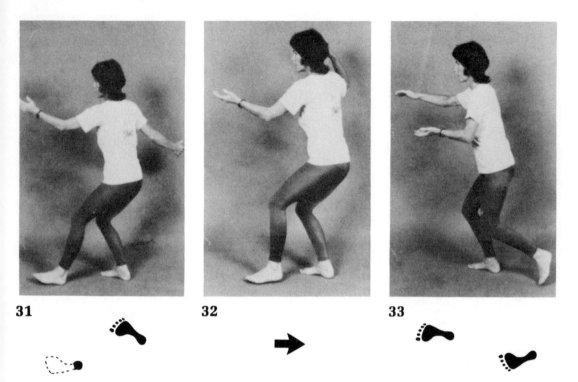

31   **32**   **33**

**6.
Reverse
Unfolding of
the Arms—
Left and Right**

1. Torso turns to the right. The right hand turns over (palm up and describes an arc) **back down across the turned body and up to the rear to be level with the shoulder,** arm slightly bent **(photo 31).** (Meanwhile the left hand immediately turns palm up.) (Moving with the turning of the body, the gaze first turns to the right then focuses ahead on the left hand.)

2. The left leg lifts very lightly and **retreats a step to left rear (photo 32), the sole of the foot touching the ground first,** then the whole foot slowly treading down. **Weight transfers to the left leg** (left hollow step) **(photo 33)** (the right foot swivelling on the ball of the foot with the turning of the body).

At the same time the right arm bends at the elbow and **changes direction to push forward,** hand passing to the front alongside the ear, (palm forward). **The left arm,** (hand palm up) bends at the elbow and then **draws back down alongside the left ribs (photo 32).**

(Gaze on right hand.)

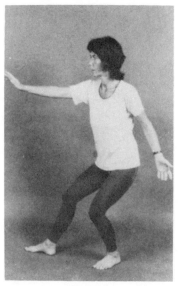
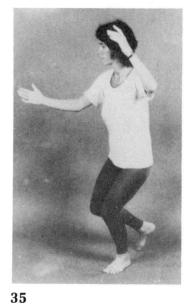
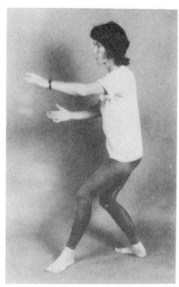

34   **35**   **36**

3. Torso turns slightly to the left.
At the same time the left hand, (palm up) **follows the turning of the body to describe an arc up to the rear** (and the right hand immediately turns palm up) **(photo 34).**
(Moving with the turning of the body, gaze first turns to the left then focuses on the right hand in front.)
4. The right leg lifts very lightly and **retreats a step to right rear (photo 35), the sole of the foot touching the ground first,** then the whole foot slowly treading down. **Weight transfers to the right leg** (right hollow step) **(photo 36),** (the left foot swivelling on the ball of the foot with the turning of the body).
At the same time the left arm bends at the elbow and **changes direction to push forward (photo 35),** hand passing to the front alongside the ear, (palm forward). **The right arm,** (hand palm up) bends at the elbow and **draws back (photo 35) down alongside the right ribs (photo 36).**
(Gaze on left hand.)
Direction: east, moving backwards to the west

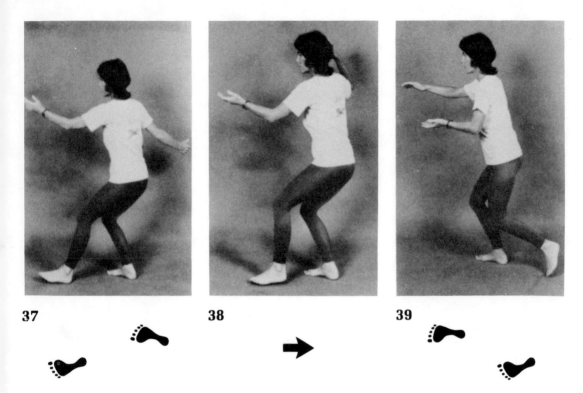

37   38   39

**6.
Reverse
Unfolding of
the Arms—
Left and Right**
continued

5. and 6. These movements are exactly the same as **Reverse Unfolding of the Arms (1) and (2) (photos 37, 38, 39).**

7. and 8. These movements are exactly the same as **Reverse Unfolding of the Arms (3) and (4) (photos 40, 41, 42).**

Direction: east, moving backwards to the west

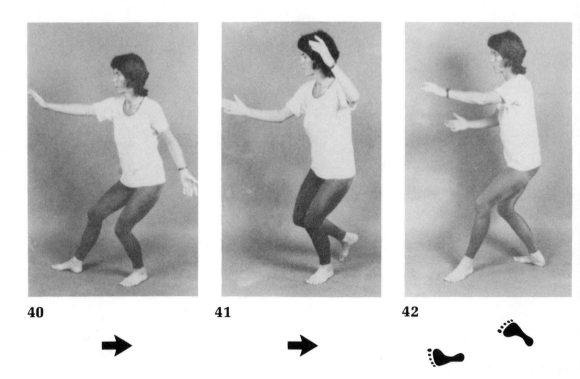

40   **41**   **42**

The hand pushing forward should not be stiff, nor should the withdrawing hand pull straight back: they both trace an arc with the turning of the body. (When pushing forward, the small of the back turns and the groin is relaxed.) Both hands move at the same pace, avoiding rigidity. (So that the feet do not tread directly behind each other, step a little to the left when stepping back with the left foot and a little to the right when stepping back with the right foot. When the right foot retreats the last time, the toes should point to the side at a somewhat greater angle in order to make easier the transition to **Grasping the Peacock's Tail**).

c

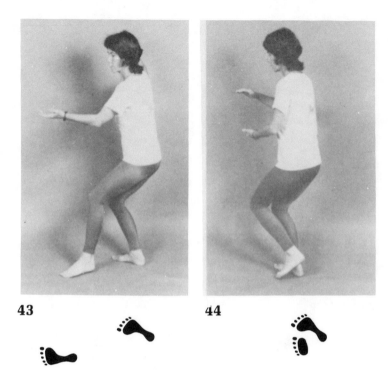

43   44

Section 3

7.
Grasping
the Peacock's
Tail—Left

1. Torso turns slightly to the right (photo 43).
At the same time the right hand (palm up) **describes an arc back and up to the rear.** (The left hand immediately turns palm up) **(photo 43).**
(Gaze on left hand.)
2. Body continues turning to the right. **Weight falls back on to the right leg and the left foot comes in to the right instep,** toes touching the ground **(photo 44).**
At the same time the left hand (palm up) **drops down across** in front of the body, (arcing up) **to the right ribs. The right arm** bends, (turning palm down) and **comes in to the right breast,** the two hands poised as if holding a balloon **(photo 44).**
(Gaze on right hand.)

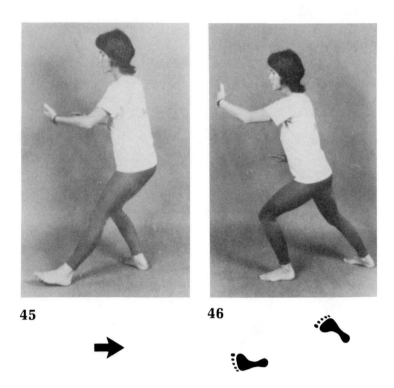

45   46

3. Torso turns slightly to the left and **the left leg steps out forward to the left (photo 45).** Torso continues turning to the left, right leg straightens as the left leg bends at the knee **to form a left bow step (photo 46).**
At the same time the left arm (palm facing rear) **draws out forward (photo 45)** and to the left, (i.e. the left arm forms a bow shape, with the outer forearm and the back of the hand pushing forward), **until it is level with the left shoulder (photo 46). The right hand drops down (photo 45) to be level with the right groin** (palm down and fingers pointing forward) **(photo 46).**
(Gaze on left forearm.)
Direction: east

(When drawing the left arm forward, an arc shape is maintained by both arms. The three actions of separating the hands, relaxing the small of the back and bowing the leg are all carried out together. In this bow step, the distance sideways between the heels should not exceed 10 cm.)

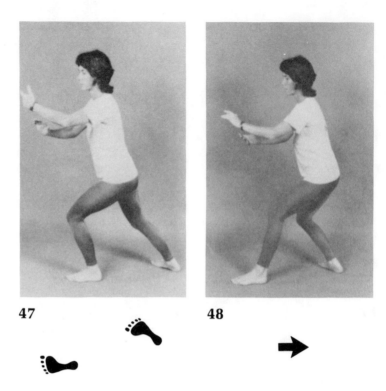

47   48

**7.
Grasping
the Peacock's
Tail—Left**
continued

Although the weight of the body is twice shifted from the left leg to the right and then back to the left during movements 4-7, the feet do not move, but remain throughout in the position shown in photo 46.

4. (Body turns slightly to the left.) **The left hand** (immediately extends forward a little) and **flips over** palm down, **while the right hand** flips over palm up, **passing forward and up in front of the body until it is under the left forearm (photo 47). Then both hands stroke downwards and backwards (photo 48),** i.e. torso turns right and the hands travel (in an arc) in front of the body down to the right rear, **until the right hand** (palm up) **is level with the right shoulder (photo 49) and the left arm** (palm facing rear) **is in front of the chest (photo 49).** (Both arms follow an arced path with the swivelling of the body.)

At the same time weight transfers on to the right leg and the left foot remains flat on the ground (photo 49). When stroking downwards and backwards, torso should not lean forward nor should the buttocks protrude.

(Gaze on right hand.)

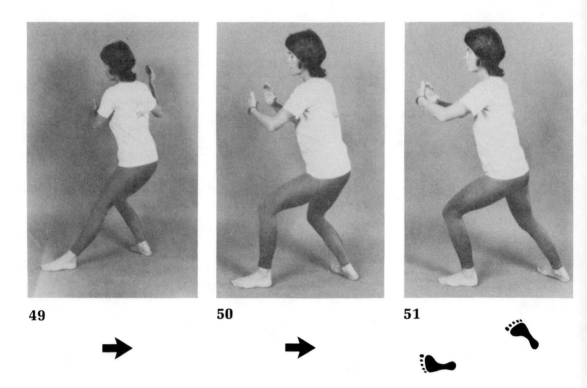

49   50   51

5. Torso turns slightly to the left. **The right arm** bends at the elbow and **changes direction** so that the right hand **comes forward to** within 5 cm of **the inner wrist of the left hand (photo 50).** Torso continues turning to the left and **both hands simultaneously slowly crowd forward,** (palm of the left hand facing the rear, palm of the right facing forward and the left forearm forming a semicircle) **(photo 51).** The torso should remain erect as it turns.

At the same time weight gradually shifts forward to form a left bow step (photo 51) (the left leg bowing and the small of the back relaxing simultaneously).

(Gaze on left wrist.)

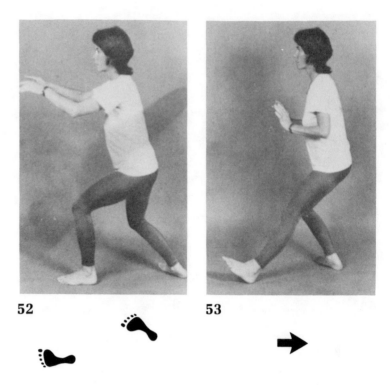

52   53

**7.
Grasping
the Peacock's
Tail—Left**
continued

6. The left hand turns palm down and **the right hand** palm down **moves forward and to the right over the top of the left wrist until both hands are at shoulder level (photo 52),** shoulder width apart. Then the right leg bends at the knee, **torso slowly sits back, weight transfers back on to the right leg and the toes of the left foot lift up (photo 53).**

At the same time both hands retract with elbows bent **to in front of the diaphragm** (palms facing forward but slightly down) **(photo 53).**

(Gaze straight ahead.)

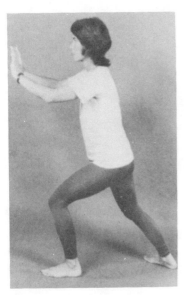

54

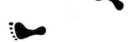

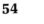

7. Without stopping at all, **weight slowly shifts forward while simultaneously both hands press forward and up,** (palms facing forward) **(photo 54).** (Both hands trace a curve, wrists at shoulder height, elbows slightly bent.) Bowed left leg in front becomes a **left bow step (photo 54).**
(Gaze straight ahead.)
Direction: east

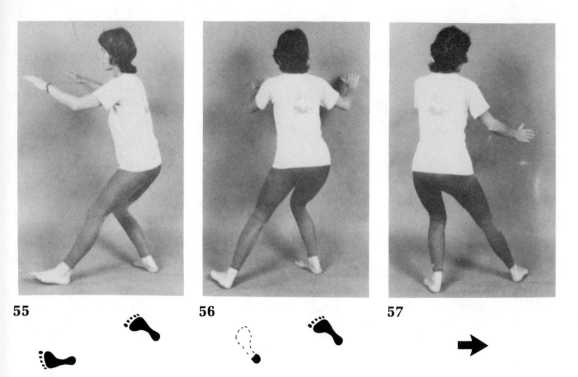

55   56   57

**8.
Grasping the
Peacock's
Tail—Right**

1. Torso sits back while also turning to the right **(photo 55).
Weight transfers on to the right leg and the toes of the left foot lift
and hook inwards (photo 56). Weight then shifts back on to the
left leg (photos 57 and 58) and the right foot comes in to the left
instep,** toes touching the ground **(photo 59).**

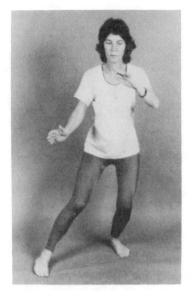 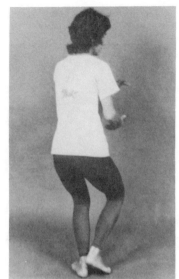

58   (reverse view to   **59**
indicate positioning
of hands)

At the same time the right hand travels to the right (in a slight
arc) still **at shoulder height** till it is outside the right shoulder
(photo 56), then (describes an arc) **down in front** of the body and
up **to the left ribs** (palm up) **(photo 59). The left hand also
remains at shoulder height (photos 57 and 58) and moves in to in
front of the left breast (photo 59)** so that the left hand (palm
down) is above the right hand, the two poised as if holding a
balloon.
(Gaze on left hand.)

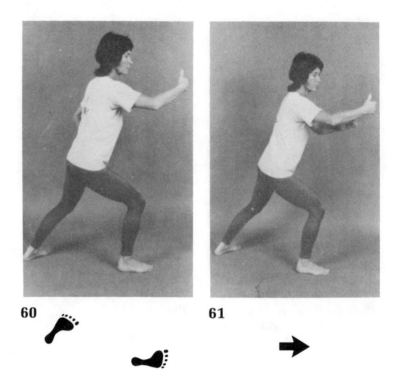

60   61

8.
Grasping
the Peacock's
Tail—Right
continued

The rest of this movement is a mirror image of **Grasping the Peacock's Tail—Left (3-7):**
2. Torso turns slightly to the right and **the right leg steps out forward to the right.** Torso continues turning to the right, left leg straightens as the right leg bends at the knee **to form a right bow step (photo 60).**
At the same time the right arm (palm facing rear) **draws out forward** and to the right **until it is level with the right shoulder. The left hand drops down to be level with the left groin** (palm down and fingers pointing forward) **(photo 60).**
(Gaze on right forearm.)
3. (Body turns slightly to the right.) **The right hand** (immediately extends forward a little) and **flips over (photo 61)** palm down, **while the left hand** flips over palm up, **passing forward and up** in front of the body **until it is under the right forearm (photo 61). Then both hands stroke downwards and backwards until the left hand** (palm up) **is level with the left shoulder and the right arm** (palm facing rear) **is in front of the chest (photo 62).**

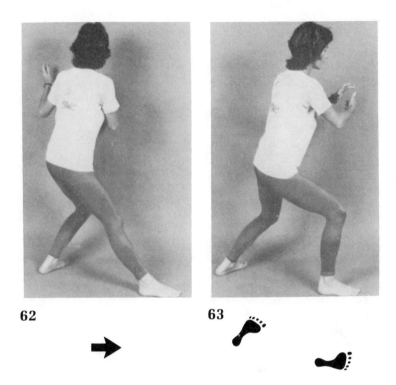

62

63

At the same time weight transfers on to the left leg and the right foot remains flat on the ground (photo 62).
(Gaze on left hand.)
4. Torso turns slightly to the right. **The left arm** bends at the elbow and **changes direction** so that the left hand **comes forward to** within 5 cm of **the inner wrist of the right hand.** Torso continues turning to the right and **both hands simultaneously slowly crowd forward,** (palm of the right hand facing the rear, palm of the left facing forward and the right forearm forming a semi-circle) **(photo 63).**
At the same time weight gradually shifts forward to form a right bow step (photo 63).
(Gaze on right wrist.)

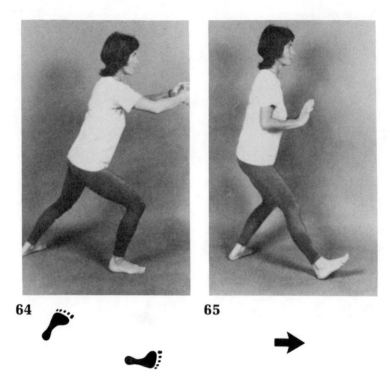

64   65

8.
Grasping
the Peacock's
Tail—Right
continued

5. The right hand turns palm down and **the left hand** palm down **moves forward and to the left over the top of the right wrist until both hands are shoulder level (photo 64),** shoulder width apart. Then the left leg bends at the knee, **torso slowly sits back, weight transfers back on to the left leg and the toes of the right foot lift up (photo 65).**
At the same time both hands retract with elbows bent **to in front of the diaphragm,** (palms facing forward but slightly down) **(photo 65).**
(Gaze straight ahead.)

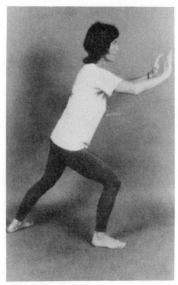

66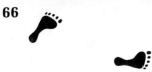

6. Without stopping at all, **weight slowly shifts forward while simultaneously both hands press forward and up,** (palms facing forward). Bowed right leg in front becomes a **right bow step (photo 66).**
(Gaze straight ahead.)
Direction: west

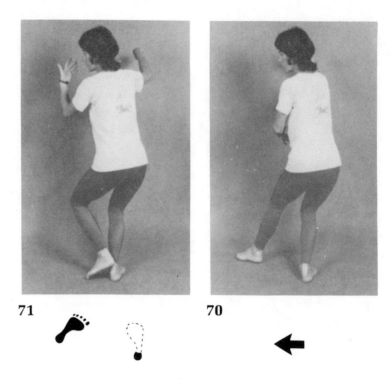

71   70

Section 4

**9.
Single Whip**

1. Torso sits back then **turns to the left. Weight slowly shifts on
to the left leg (photo 67), the right toes lift up and hook inwards,
heel remaining on the ground (photo 68).**
As the torso turns, the hands travel (on an arced path) to the left.
The left hand (palm facing left) **stays in front of the left shoulder
as the body turns (photo 68). The right hand drops down (photo
67),** passing in front of the body **across to the left ribs,** (palm
facing down then obliquely upwards) **(photo 68).**
(Gaze on left hand.)

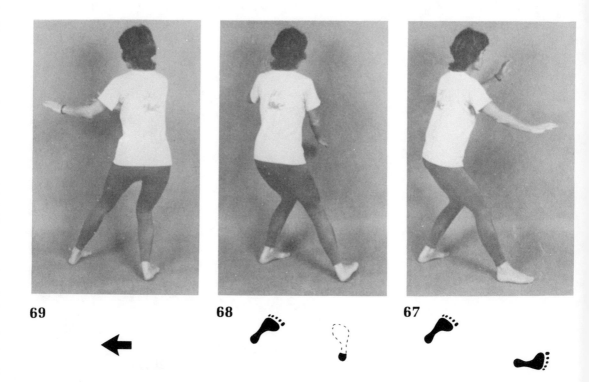

69

68

67

2. Weight slowly shifts back on to the right leg (and torso starts to turn to the right) **(photo 69). The left foot moves in to the right instep,** toes touching the ground **(photo 71).**
At the same time the right hand (describes an arc) **back up past the right shoulder (photo 69) then out away from the body** at an angle **to come to rest at shoulder height** with the hand changed into a hook **(photo 71). The left hand arcs down and to the right (photo 69)** across the body **(photo 70)** then up **until it is in front of the right shoulder,** (palm facing inwards) **(photo 71).**
(Gaze on left hand.)

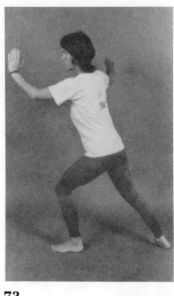

73

9.
Single Whip
continued

3. Torso turns slightly to the left, the left foot steps out forward and to the left **(photo 72)** and the right leg straightens as the left leg bows **and weight moves forward to make a left bow step (photo 73).**

As the weight moves forward, **the left hand moves with the body, slowly turning** palm forward **(photo 72) to push out in front of the left shoulder,** fingers at eye level and arm a little bent **(photo 73).**

(Gaze on left hand.)

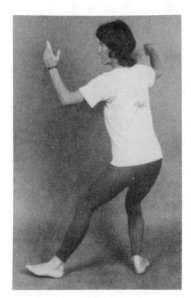

72

Direction: very slightly south of east
Torso is erect (and the small of the back relaxed). In the completed bow step, the right elbow hangs down (the left elbow is above the left knee and both shoulders are heavy). The left hand turns gradually palm forward as torso turns, not quickly or at the last minute.

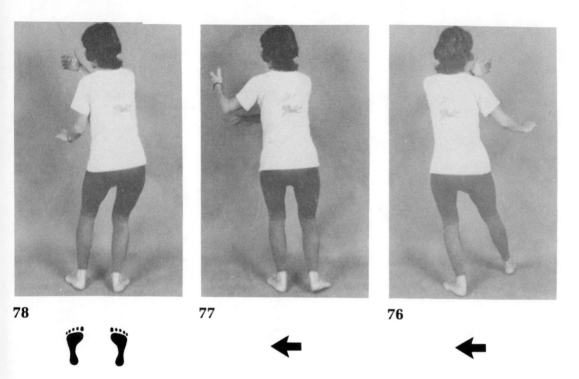

78   **77**   **76**

10.
Cloud Hands

1. Weight shifts back on to the right leg (photo 74), torso turns right and **the left toes lift up and hook inwards, heel remaining on the ground (photo 75).**
At the same time the left hand (describes an arc) **down (photo 74) then to the right across the body and up to the right shoulder** (the same movement as in **Single Whip (2)** (palm facing obliquely backwards) **(photo 75).** The right hand changes back to an opened hand, (palm facing forward right) **(photo 75).** (Gaze on left hand.)

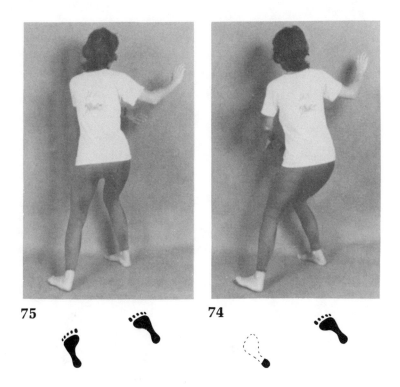

75   74

2. **As torso slowly turns left, weight slowly returns to the left leg (photo 76). Then the right foot moves to the left, parallel with the left foot (photo 78)** (coming to rest on the ground 10-20 cm to the right of the left foot).

At the same time the left hand (palm facing inwards) **passes from right to left (photo 77) in front of the face. The right hand drops down (photo 76) then passes** (in a slight arc) **across the body (photo 77) from right to left and back up until it is in front of the left shoulder,** (palm facing obliquely backwards) **(photo 78).**

(Gaze on left hand.)

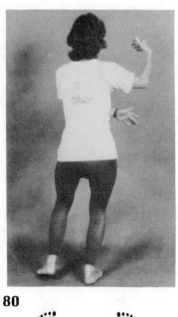

80

10.
Cloud Hands
continued

3. (Torso turns slightly to the right,) **weight shifts on to the right leg (photo 79) and the left leg steps out sideways in a crab-like step (photo 80).**

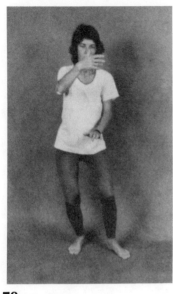

(reverse view to
indicate positioning
of hands)

79

**At the same time the left hand drops down and passes across in
front of the body from left to right (photo 79)** then arcs **up until it
is in front of the right shoulder,** (palm facing obliquely backwards) **(photo 80). The right hand** (palm facing inwards) **passes
from left to right in front of the face (photo 80).**
(Gaze on right hand.)
Direction: south

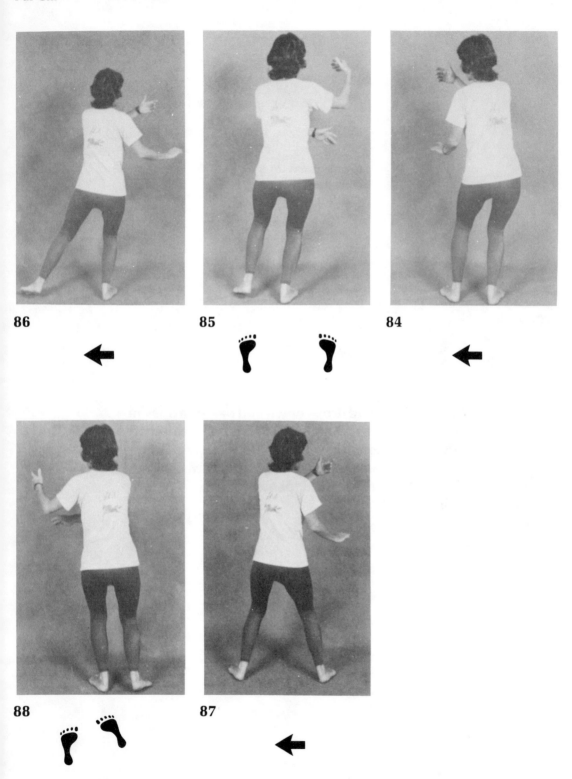

86

85

84

88

87

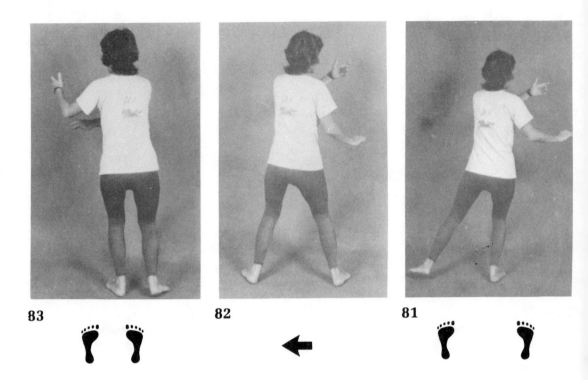

83   82   ←   81

4. and 5. These movements are exactly the same as **Cloud Hands** **(2 and 3) (photos 81, 82, 83, 84, 85).**
6. This movement is exactly the same as **Cloud Hands (2)** **(photos 86, 87, 88).**
Direction: south

10.
Cloud Hands
continued

(The fulcrum on which the body turns is the small of the back; hips are relaxed) and you should avoid bobbing up and down. Shoulders turn smoothly and evenly with the body. **As you step sideways the ball of the foot touches the ground first,** with toes pointing forward. (Eyes focus on and follow whichever hand is passing across the face. On the third **Cloud Hands,** hook the right heel inwards a little in order to make easier the transition to the **Single Whip** which follows.)

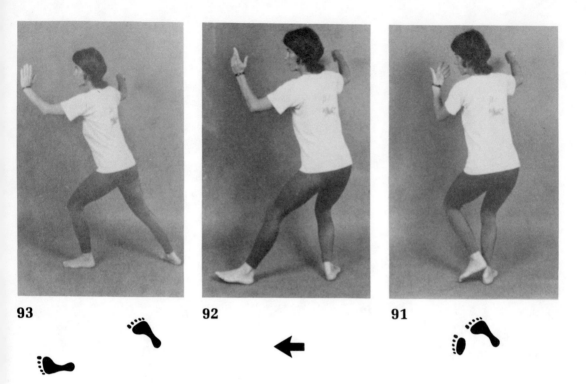

93　　　　　　　　　　**92**　　　　　　　　**91**

11.
Single Whip

This movement is exactly the same as **9. Single Whip (2 and 3)** **(photos 89, 90, 91, 92, 93)**.

Direction: very slightly south of east

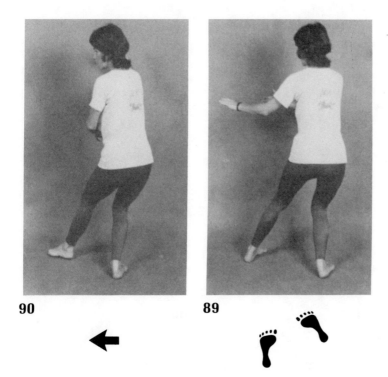

90

89

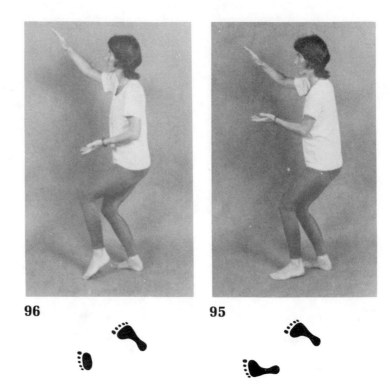

96　　　　　　　**95**

Section 5

12.
Testing the
High Horse

1. Weight transfers wholly on the front (left) foot. The right foot takes a half step forward (photo 94) then weight goes back on to the right leg (as torso turns to the right a little) and the left heel begins to leave the ground **(photo 95).**

At the same time the hooked right hand opens out and **the palms of both hands turn in to face each other,** elbows remaining bent **(photo 94).**

(Gaze straight ahead, a little to the left.)

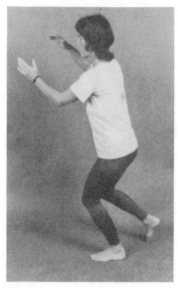

94

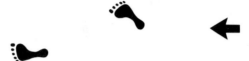

2. (Torso turns a little to the left so that you are facing straight forward.) **The left foot moves forward a little, toes barely touching the ground** (left heel stance) **(photo 96).**
At the same time the right hand (palm facing forward) **pushes forward at eye level** alongside the right ear. **The left hand pulls back in** (palm up) **to alongside the left waist (photo 96)**.
(Gaze on right hand.)
Direction: east

Torso should be erect (shoulders heavy and the right elbow hanging down a little). Avoid bobbing up and down as weight shifts from foot to foot.

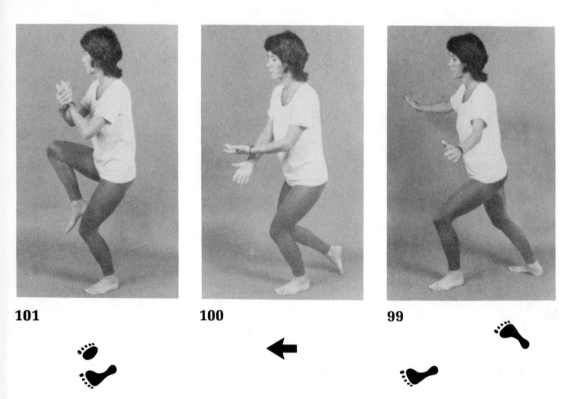

101   100   99

**13.
Planting the
Foot—Right**

1. The left leg lifts forward to the outside left (toes hooked out slightly) **(photo 98), weight shifts forward** and the right leg straightens **to make a left bow step (photo 99).**

At the same time the left hand (palm up) **comes forward and up to above the right wrist** (crossed wrists) **(photo 97)** then turns palm down. **Both hands then separate away from each other (photo 98) and down** as if caressing the outside of a balloon **(photo 99).**

(Gaze straight ahead.)

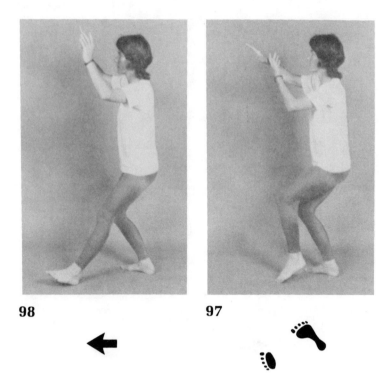

98   **97**

2. Weight transfers wholly on to the left leg and the right leg moves forward (photo 100) to the left instep, toes touching the ground.

At the same time both hands meet and cross, (right hand underneath,) at the bottom of the balloon **(photo 100) then lift up together,** crossed and (with the right hand outside), **to the centre of the chest** (palms facing backwards) **(photo 101).**

(Gaze forward, a little to the right.)

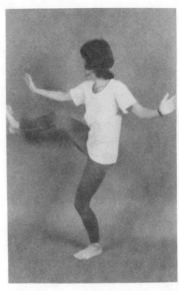

103

**13.
Planting the
Foot—Right**
continued

3. The right knee lifts up (photo 102) then the right foot slowly kicks out to the right at an angle of about 30° from straight ahead **(photo 103).**
At the same time both hands turn (palms forward) as the **arms separate (photo 102) and reach out to form a straight line with the shoulders,** elbows bent a little **(photo 103).**
(Gaze on right hand.)
Direction: almost south-east

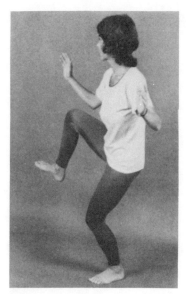

102

Torso should be erect. (Wrists are level with the shoulders as the arms separate.) Kick out with the heel of the right leg and keep the left leg bent. (The kick and the separating of the hands take place together.) The right arm should extend along the top of the right leg.

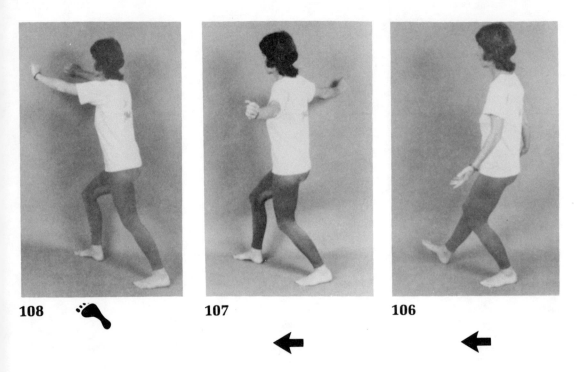

108   107   106

14.
Twin Peaks
Piercing
the Ears

1. The right knee stays up as the right foot and lower leg drop back to hang straight down from the knee (photo 104).
At the same time the left hand moves forward over the shoulder (and both hands turn palm up as the left hand comes level with the right) **(photo 104). Both hands then continue in an arc down in front of the body to pass on either side of the raised right knee.** (Gaze straight ahead.)
2. The right foot drops forward (photo 106) to the right and **weight slowly shifts forward on to it (photo 107) to make a right bow step (photo 108).**

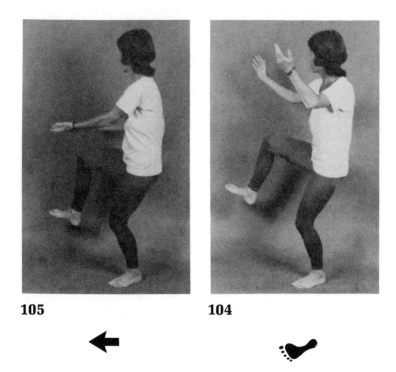

105   **104**

At the same time both hands continue on their downward and
backward arc, slowly forming into fists. The hands go back past
the hips (photo 106) then arc up and forward past the shoulders
(photo 107) to come to rest level with each other at ear level in
front of the face (photo 108). (The eyes of the fists (thumb side)
point in towards each other and slightly down, 10-20 cm apart.)
(Gaze on right fist.)
Direction: almost south-east

(Neck should remain erect, the small of the back and hips
relaxed, shoulders heavy and elbows hanging down. Both arms
maintain an arc shape during their travel. Heels should be about
10 cm apart sideways.)

D

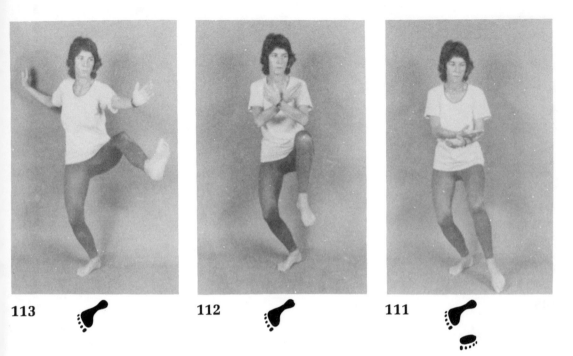

113   **112**   **111**

15.
Revolving
Planting the
Foot—Left

1. The left knee bends and **weight is pulled back on to the left leg. Torso turns to the left and the right heel remains on the ground as the toes of the right foot lift and hook inwards (photo 109). At the same time both** fists revert to open **hands, separating out and away from each other** (palms facing forward) **(photo 109).** (Gaze on left hand.)

2. Weight shifts back on to the right leg (photo 110) and the left foot comes in to the right instep (photo 111), toes touching the ground.

At the same time both hands continue separating away from each other and down (photo 110) as if caressing the outside of a balloon, cross (with the left hand underneath) at the bottom of the balloon **(photo 111) then lift up together,** still crossed (and with the left hand outside,) **to the centre of the chest,** (palms facing backwards) **(photo 112).**

(Gaze to the left.)

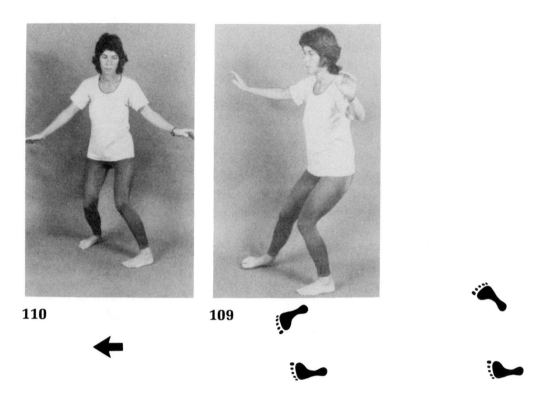

110   109

3. This movement mirrors **Planting the Foot—Right (3)**:
The left knee lifts up, then the left foot slowly kicks out to the left
at an angle of about 30° from straight ahead **(photo 113).**
At the same time both hands turn (palms forward) as the **arms**
separate and reach out to form a straight line with the shoulders,
elbows bent a little **(photo 113).**
(Gaze on left hand.)
Direction: almost north-west

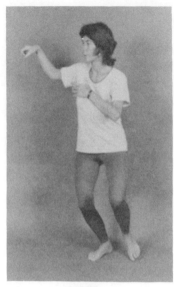

114

Section 6

16.
Low Free
Standing—
Left

1. The left foot and lower leg drop back down, not quite touching the ground, **as torso turns to the right (photo 114).**
At the same time the right hand changes into a hook and **pulls a little closer in to the right shoulder, while the left hand arcs,** (up), **back,** (then down slightly) **to come to rest in front of the right shoulder,** (palm facing obliquely backwards) **(photo 114).**
(Gaze on right hand.)
Direction in this position is north
2. The right leg slowly bends down as far as possible and the left leg extends out sideways to the left. Do not tip the body forward as you squat down. **Weight remains wholly on the bent right leg** (attacking step) **(photo 115).** (The left toes hook inwards as the left leg extends, and the soles of both feet should be on the ground. The left toes step out in a direct line with the right heel.)
At the same time the left hand, (thumb leading the palm to turn outwards,) **falls down to the left** (skirting along the inside of the outstretched left leg) **(photo 115).**
(Gaze on left hand.)

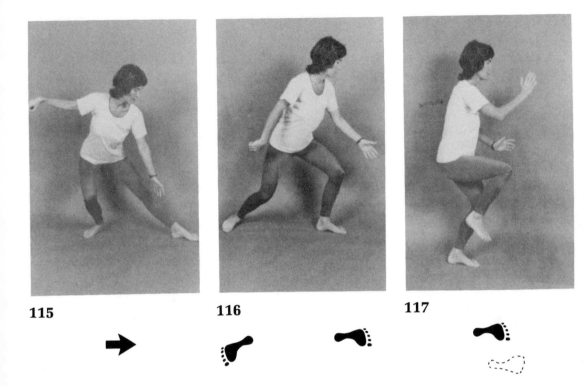

115   116   117

3. Weight shifts forward (and, with the left heel acting as the pivot, the left toes turn out a little). **The left leg bows forward while the right leg lingers where it was** and **torso** simultaneously **veers left** and lifts forward **(photo 116)**.

At the same time the left hand continues forward and up, (palm facing right,) **while the right hooked hand falls** (with the hook trailing behind) **(photo 116)**.

(Gaze on left hand.)

4. As the entire weight of the body falls on to the left leg, the right foot slowly pulls forward and up to make a left free standing step (one-legged stance) **(photo 117)**.

At the same time the hooked right hand opens out into a hand, **arcing forward and up,** (travelling outside and with the lifting right leg,) **to come to rest elbow over the right knee** (palm facing left). **Left hand falls back to the left hip,** (palm down and fingers pointing ahead) **(photo 117)**.

(Gaze on right hand.)

Direction: west

Torso remains erect, left leg remains bent and the toes of the raised right leg hang downwards easily.

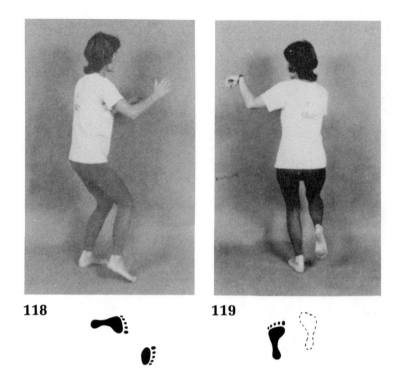

118   **119**

**17.
Low Free
Standing—
Right**

**1. The ball of the right foot comes down to touch the ground in
front of the left foot (photo 118)** then, **swivelling on the ball of the
left foot, the left heel moves to turn the whole body to the left,** i.e.
now facing south (photo 119).
At the same time the left hand moves back and up **to outside the
left shoulder,** changing into a hook. **The right hand arcs** with the
turning of the body **back across to come to rest in front of the left
shoulder** (palm facing obliquely backwards) **(photo 119).**
(Gaze on left hand.)
This position is a mirror image of **Low Free Standing—Left (1).**
The rest of this movement is a mirror image of **Low Free
Standing—Left (2-4):**
**2. The left leg slowly bends down as far as possible and the right
leg extends out sideways to the right. Weight remains wholly on
the bent left leg (photo 120).**
At the same time the right hand, (thumb leading the palm to turn
outwards,) **falls down to the right** (skirting along the inside of
the outstretched right leg) **(photo 120).**
(Gaze on right hand.)

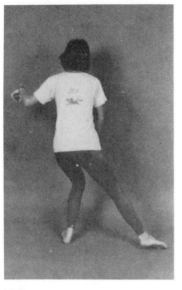
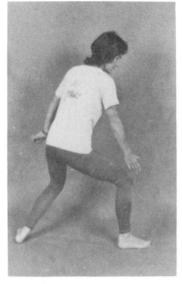
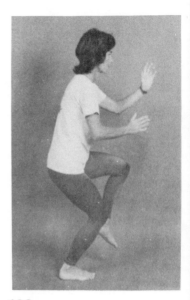

120   **121**   **122**

3. Weight shifts forward (and, with the right heel acting as the pivot, the right toes turn out a little). **The right leg bows forward while the left leg lingers where it was and torso** simultaneously **veers right** and lifts forward **(photo 121)**.

At the same time the right hand continues forward and up, (palm facing left,) **while the left hooked hand falls** (with the hook trailing behind) **(photo 121)**.

(Gaze on right hand.)

4. As the entire weight of the body falls on to the right leg, the left foot slowly pulls forward and up to make a right free standing step (photo 122).

At the same time the hooked left hand opens out into a hand, **arcing forward and up,** (travelling outside and with the lifting left leg,) **to come to rest elbow over the left knee** (palm facing right). **Right hand falls back to the right hip** (palm down and fingers pointing ahead) **(photo 122)**.

(Gaze on left hand.)

Direction: west

After the ball of the right foot touches the ground, it lifts up a fraction before reaching out sideways to the right.

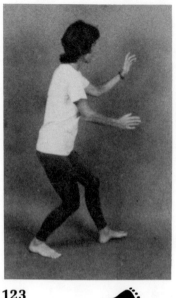

123

Section 7

**18.
Piercing
the Shuttle**

1. Torso turns slightly to the left, **left foot steps forward and to the left** with the toes hooked outwards and the right heel lifts off the ground; both knees are bent **(photo 123). Then the right foot comes in to the left instep,** toes touching the ground **(photo 124). At the same time both hands pull in to in front of the chest (photo 123)**, (palms facing each other) and **left above the right,** poised as if they were holding a balloon **(photo 124).**
(Gaze on left forearm.)
2. Body turns to the right, **the right leg steps out forward to the right (photo 125)** and bows to **make a right bow step (photo 126).**

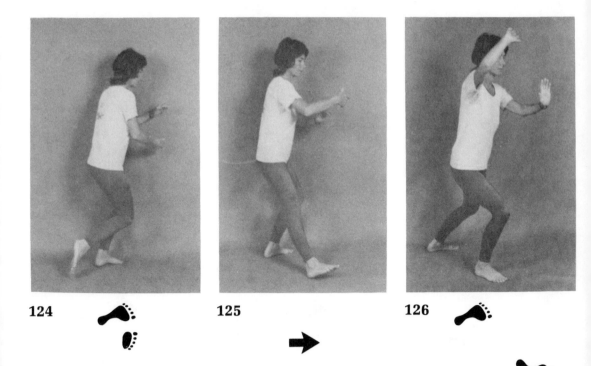

124   125   126

At the same time the right hand arcs up (in front of the face) **(photo 125)** (as it turns over) **to come to rest** (palm up) **above the right temple (photo 126). The left hand pulls in** and down to the left **(photo 125), then pushes out forward in front of the body to come to rest at nose level** (palm forward) **(photo 126).**
(Gaze on left hand.)
Direction: almost north-west

Don't lean forward as the left hand pushes forward. Avoid hunching the right shoulder as the right hand lifts up. (The bowing forward with the right leg and the motions of the hands all take place together. Heels in this bow step should be about 30 cm apart, sideways.)

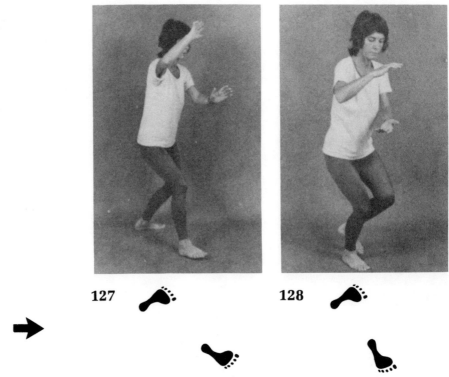

127   128

18.
Piercing
the Shuttle
continued

3. Weight shifts backwards a fraction (photo 127) to allow the right toes to lift up and hook out slightly, **then weight immediately transfers back on to the right leg. The left foot then moves up to the right instep,** toes touching the ground **(photo 128).**
At the same time both hands pull in in front of the chest, (palms facing each other) and **right above the left,** poised as if holding a balloon **(photo 128).**
(Gaze on right forearm.)

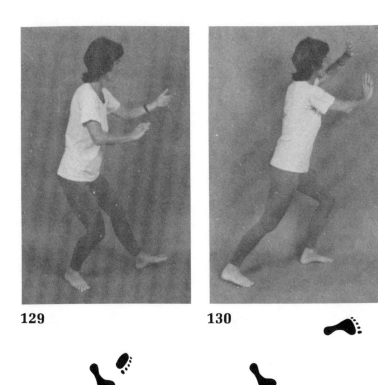

129   130

4. This movement is a mirror image of **Piercing the Shuttle (2):**
Body turns to the left, **the left leg steps out forward to the left
(photo 129)** and bows **to make a left bow step (photo 130).
At the same time the left hand arcs up** (in front of the face **(photo
129)** as it turns over) **to come to rest** (palm up) **above the left
temple (photo 130). The right hand pulls in** and down to the right
**(photo 129) then pushes out forward in front of the body to come
to rest at nose level** (palm forward) **(photo 130).**
(Gaze on right hand.)
Direction: almost south-west

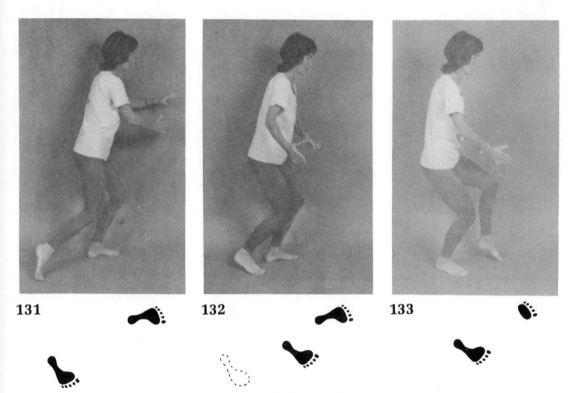

131   132   133

**19.
Needle
Pointing to the
Bottom of the
Sea**

Weight is taken wholly by the left leg (photo 131) then, (as torso turns a little to the right,) **the right foot takes a half step forward (photo 132). Weight then transfers back on to the right foot and the left foot moves forward a little,** toes touching the ground (left heel stance) **(photo 133).**

At the same time the right hand draws back, **down** and across the body **(photo 132) then up until it is level with the right ear. It then** moves with the body as the body turns left, **piercing down diagonally forward to knee level** (palm facing left and fingers pointing obliquely down) **(photo 133). Meanwhile the left hand curves** out in front and down **(photo 132),** then **in to come to rest alongside the left groin** (palm down and fingers pointing ahead) **(photo 133).**

(Gaze is on the ground in front of you.)

Direction: west

(Torso first turns to the right, then to the left.) Don't lean forward in this stance. Avoid lowering the head and sticking the buttocks out. Left leg remains bent.

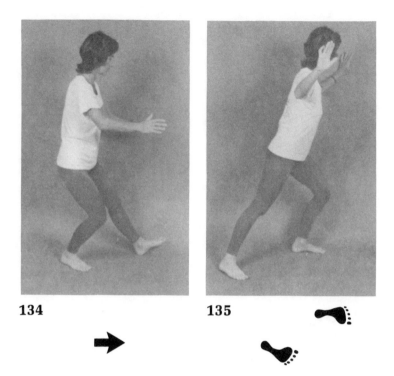

134   **135**

(Torso turns right a little) and **the left foot steps forward (photo 134)** bowing **to form a left bow step (photo 135).**
At the same time the right hand lifts up out to the right (palm turning over to face obliquely upwards,) **to come to rest above and in front of the right temple,** (thumb down). **The left hand lifts up across the chest then pushes out forward to be level with the nose** (palm facing forward) **(photo 135).**
(Gaze on left hand.)
Direction: west

**20.
Ducking
through Arms**

(Torso should be erect and the small of the back and hips relaxed.) The left arm is not fully extended and the muscles of the back feel a slight stretching. (The movements of the hands and the left leg all take place together. Heels should be about 10 cm apart, sideways.)

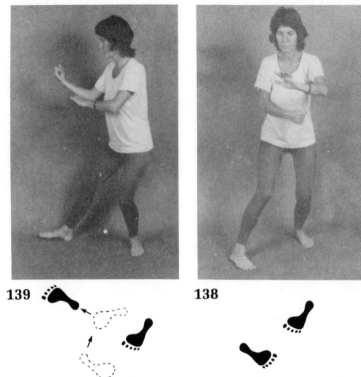

139   138

Section 8

**21.
Revolving
Block Punch**

1. Torso sits back and **weight shifts on to the right leg (photo 136) as the body turns around to the right and the toes of the left foot lift up and hook inwards** (to the right), **left heel remaining on the ground (photo 137). Then weight goes back on to the left leg (photo 138).**

At the same time the right hand arcs down and to the right **(photo 136),** forming into a fist (with the heel of the hand facing downwards,) **across the front of the waist (photo 137) and up to the left ribs (photo 138). The left hand moves to the right a little to in front of the forehead** (palm obliquely up) **(photo 137).**

(Gaze straight ahead of your turning body.)

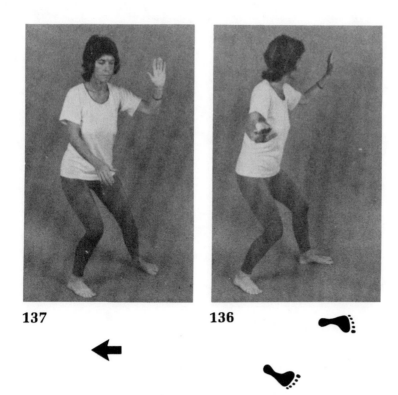

137   136

2. As the body continues turning to the right, the right foot comes back in towards the left foot (but does not hesitate or touch the ground) and immediately steps out forward with toes pointing outwards (photo 139).
At the same time the right fist (turning palm up as it moves,) passes up back across the chest towards the right (photo 139). The left hand falls down (photo 139) to pull in alongside the left hip (palm down and fingers pointing ahead).
(Gaze on right fist.)

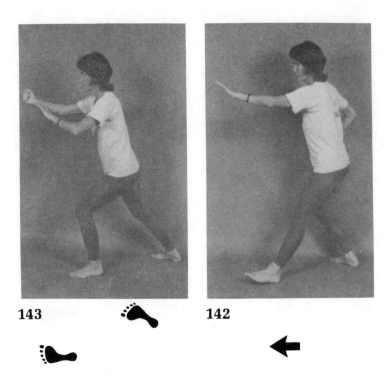

143   142

21.
Revolving
Block Punch
continued

**3. Weight moves straight on to the right leg (photo 140) and the
left leg immediately steps forward** and to the left **(photo 142).
At the same time the right fist** (palm up) **pulls** (in an arc) **back to
the right side at the waist (photos 141 and 142) while the left
hand travels up and forward** (palm facing obliquely forward)
(photo 142).
(Gaze on left hand.)

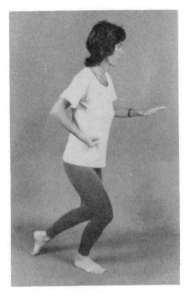

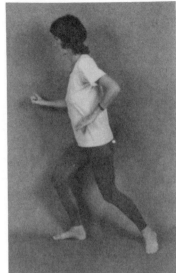

141 (reverse view to indicate positioning of hands)

140

4. The left leg bows as **weight shifts forward to make a left bow step (photo 143).**
At the same time the right fist (turning thumb up,) **punches out forward and up to chest height, and the left hand pulls back a little to come to rest alongside the inside of the right forearm (photo 143).**
(Gaze on right fist.)
Direction: east

Don't clench the right fist too tightly. (As the fist pulls back in to the waist, the forearm arcs in then out again, palm up.) As the fist punches forward, the right shoulder follows forward, shoulders heavy and elbow down, keeping a slight bend in the right arm. (In the bow step the heels should be about 10 cm apart, sideways.)

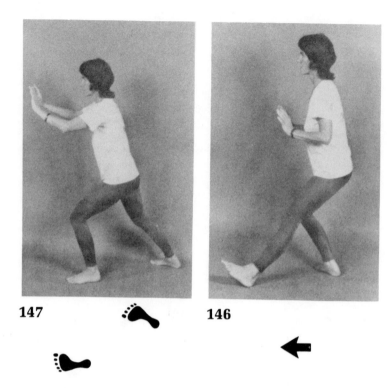

147   146

22.
As Though
Sealing Up

During this movement only the weight of the body shifts from leg to leg; the feet themselves do not move from the preceding left bow step position.

1. Body sits back as **weight transfers back on to the right leg** and the right leg bows back **with the toes of the left foot lifting up and the left leg straightening (photo 145).**

At the same time the left hand slips beneath the right wrist (photo 144), the right fist opens up into a hand **and both hands** (slowly turn palm up) as they **separate away from each other and start to pull back in towards the chest (photo 145).**

(Gaze straight ahead.)

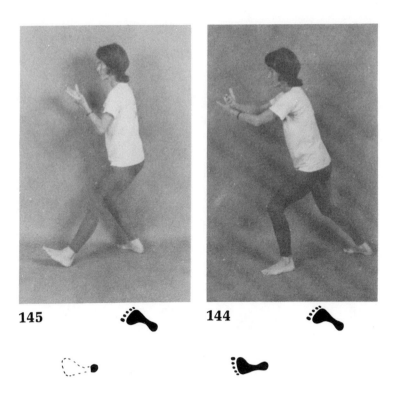

145   144

2. Weight shifts back on to the left leg and the left leg bows forward to **make a left bow step (photo 147).**
Both hands pull in towards the chest (as they simultaneously turn over palms down,) **then travel** shoulder width apart **down in front of the body to the stomach (photo 146), then push back up and out to** rest with wrists at **shoulder height** (palms facing forward) **(photo 147).**
(Gaze straight ahead.)
Direction: east

Avoid leaning backwards or sticking the buttocks out as the body sits back. (As the hands pull back in to the body, shoulders and elbows spread outwards a fraction.) Hands should not be more than shoulder width apart as they push forward.

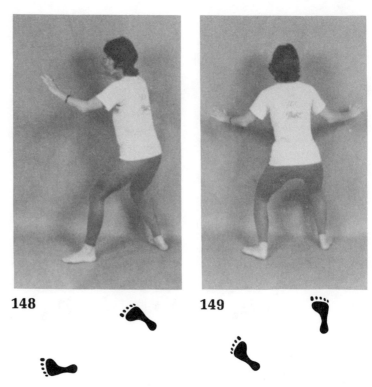

148   149

23.
Crossed Hands

1. As both knees bend, **weight moves largely on to the right leg, the toes of the left foot lift up** (heel remaining on the ground) **and the body turns to the right.** While the body swivels round to the right, **the toes of the right foot also swivel a little out to the right (photo 148).**

At the same time the right hand travels to the right with the body (arcing across and out) to be **level with the left hand, which remains in front of the left shoulder.** (Both palms face forward) and elbows are bent **(photo 148).**

(Gaze on right hand.)

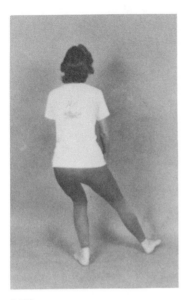

150

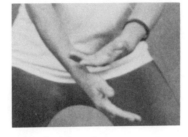

(Detail of hands in
Photo 150)

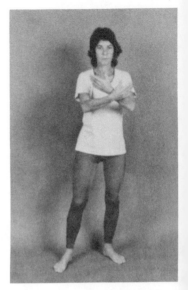

151   (reverse view to
indicate positioning
of hands)

2. Weight slowly goes back on to the left leg as the toes of the
right foot hook in **(photo 149). Then straight away the right foot
steps in sideways to come to rest shoulder width from the left,**
toes pointing straight ahead and **weight is taken equally by both
legs as they slowly straighten (photo 151).**
At the same time both hands arc down as though caressing a
very large balloon **(photo 149), meet and cross** (with the right
hand underneath) in front of the abdomen **(photo 150) and lift up
together in front of the chest until wrists are level with the
shoulders** (palms facing backwards) **(photo 151).**
(Gaze straight ahead.)
Direction: south

Don't lean forward as the hands descend and rise. On standing
upright, the body should be erect, (with suspended crown. Arms
are gently rounded throughout this movement, shoulders heavy
and elbows hanging).

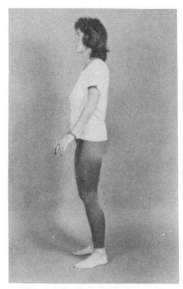

(side view to
indicate positioning
of hands)

152

**24.
Gathering In**

Hands separate as they turn over palms down **and arms slowly fall down to come to rest on either side of the body (photo 152).** (Gaze straight ahead.)
Direction: south

Keep the whole body relaxed as the hands separate and fall, and allow *ch'i* to sink slowly to the *tan t'ien*. When your breathing returns to normal, bring your left foot in alongside the right and rest for a few moments.

PART 3
PRINCIPLES IN PRACTICE

7. Coordinating Breathing With Postures

An integral part of the practice of t'ai chi is regulating breathing and bodily movements in such a way that the two flow together easily, rhythmically and harmoniously, and once you are familiar with the whole cycle you can start to work on this aspect.

However, coordinating breathing and postures is not just a matter of inhaling deeply as you start to move out of a posture and exhaling as you reach the next posture. Some movements, e.g. *Stroking the Wild Horse's Mane, Crane's Wings, Brushing the Knee Twist*, are executed to a single complete breath while others are not, e.g. *Grasping the Peacock's Tail, Single Whip*. Whether a movement is executed to one complete breath or to two or three depends on the role of that movement in the martial arts.

The general principle can be summarised as **rise on inhalation and fall on exhalation; close on inhalation and open on exhalation.** Inhalation takes place on the defensive movements of hoarding, closing and changing, while exhalation takes place on the attacking movements of releasing, opening and striking. Breathing thus flows together very naturally with the movements. Shortness of breath or a feeling of suffocation prevents the full focusing of strength, and harmonising breathing and movements prevents shortness of breath.

Since the movements joining postures to each other also derive from the martial arts, these too are coordinated with breathing on the same principle of defence-attack as with the actual postures.

The following postures, taken from the 88-posture Yang style t'ai chi widely practised on mainland China at present, are illustrated to show the general principle of blending breathing with movements as it relates to defence (changing) and attack (striking). Since the emphasis here is on the principles of breathing, only the major bodily movements will be described rather than giving a detailed and precise explanation of how each part of the body moves.

A. Grasping the Peacock's Tail—Right

1. Weight on left leg; right foot with toes pointing ahead poised in front of left foot and about to step forward. Hands (palms facing each other), left above and right below, poised as if **inhale** holding a balloon in front of the chest.

Right foot steps forward and slightly to the right, heel leading. Then, as the foot touches down, right leg bows and weight shifts forward to form a right bow step. Right hand draws forward and up (palm facing in), left hand drops down and backwards to left **exhale** hip (palm down).

2. Body sits back into a right hollow stance and torso turns slightly left. Left hand moves forward and up a little, then both **inhale** hands pull back and down to the left side.

Torso turns right, right leg bows and weight shifts forward to form a right bow step. Both hands push forward, right hand in front (palm facing inwards) and left pushing palm forward until **exhale** they are shoulder height in front of the body.

3. Body sits back into a right hollow stance. Hands separate and **inhale** pull back shoulder width apart in towards the chest.

Body and weight move forward and right leg bows into a right bow step. Hands (heel of the hands leading) push back up and **exhale** forward until wrists are at shoulder height.

B. Single Whip

This posture follows on from *Grasping the Peacock's Tail* above.

1. Torso turns left as weight starts to move on to left leg. Both hands start travelling left with the body, left hand remaining in front of the left shoulder and the right starting to sweep down and to the left across the body.   **inhale**

   With weight on left leg, the toes of the right foot lift up and hook inwards (right hollow stance). Left hand continues moving with the body and the right hand starts coming up in front of the left ribs.   **exhale**

2. Torso starts to turn to the right as weight transfers to the right leg. Right hand changes direction at the left shoulder to pull back (palm facing inwards) towards the right shoulder and the left hand starts to arc down then to the right across the body. **inhale**

   Left foot moves in towards the right instep (T-step). The right hand hangs in a hook outside the right shoulder and the left hand comes up in front of right ribs until it is in front of the right shoulder (palm facing in).   **exhale**

3. Torso starts to turn to the left and the left foot steps lightly out forward to the left. The left hand changes direction at the right shoulder to pull left (palm facing inwards) across in front of the face, elbow hanging down.   **inhale**

   Left heel touches the ground, left leg bows and weight shifts forward to make a left bow step. Left hand (palm turning out) pushes out to the left to rest in front of the left shoulder above the toes of the left foot.   **exhale**

C. Raised Hands

This movement is the reverse of *Strumming the Lute*, and follows on from *Single Whip* above.

Torso sits back and starts turning right, weight shifts a little on to the right leg as the left toes lift up and hook inwards about 45°. Then weight goes back on to the left leg as the right foot lifts up and arcs in towards the left foot. Right hooked hand opens out and both hands start to pull in towards each other across the front of the body.   **inhale**

   Right heel, toes pointing up, comes to rest barely touching the ground about 40 cm in front of the left heel in a right hollow stance. Right hand comes to rest in front of the nose and above the toes of the right foot (palm in and fingers pointing obliquely upwards). Left hand comes to rest (palm in and fingers pointing obliquely upwards) in front of the left ribs and opposite the inside of the right elbow.   **exhale**

D. Crane's Wings

This movement follows on from *Raised Hands* above.

1. Weight remains on left leg as the body starts to turn left and the right foot lifts up and starts to turn inwards. Hands turn palms facing each other about 20 cm apart in a stroking motion, **inhale** right descending and left ascending.

Right foot continues turning until the toes are pointing ahead, then treads down firmly on the ground as weight is shifted gradually on to it. The hands continue their stroking motion until they are poised as if holding a balloon, left on top and right **exhale** below.

2. Torso turns a fraction to the right as the left foot lifts and comes to rest in front with toes lightly touching the ground (heel stance) and the whole body rises up imperceptibly. The left hand drops down (palm down) and the right hand comes up (palm **inhale** facing inwards) until it is about forehead level.

The body sinks imperceptibly as the left side of the chest pulls the torso slightly to the left, the muscles in the right side of the chest sink down, the right shoulder joint relaxes down, the right elbow hangs down and the left hand settles gently alongside **exhale** the left hip.

E. Brushing the Knee Twist—Left

This movement follows on from *Crane's Wings* above.

1. Torso turns slightly to the left, then back to the right. Left foot moves back to touch the ground at the right instep (T-step). The right hand drops down across the front of the body and arcs back and then up to outside and behind the right shoulder, elbow bent, hand pushing forward at ear level (palm obliquely up). Left hand comes up to shoulder level at the left, then arcs across the **inhale** body to the right breast (palm obliquely down).

2. Torso turns left, left foot steps out forward left to make a left bow step. Right hand curves past the ear and pushes forward level with the tip of the nose and the left hand drops down and brushes back from in front of the left knee to rest alongside the **exhale** left groin (fingers pointing ahead).

F. Brushing the Knee Twist—Right

This movement follows on from *Brushing the Knee Twist—Left*.

1. Right leg bends at the knee, torso sits back, weight moves on to the right leg, left toes lift up and hook out, then weight transfers wholly on to the bent left leg. Right foot comes in to the left instep, toes touching the ground (T-step). Left hand arcs back and up to outside and behind the left shoulder, elbow bent, hand pushing forward at ear level (palm obliquely up). Right hand arcs up and then down to the left to in front of the left shoulder (palm obliquely down).   **inhale**

2. Torso turns right, the right foot steps out forward right to make a right bow step. Left hand curves past the ear and pushes forward level with the tip of the nose and the right hand drops down and brushes back from in front of the right knee to rest alongside the right groin (fingers pointing ahead).   **exhale**

G. Cloud Hands

1. The left leg has reached out to the left and touched on to the ground, and weight has just transferred wholly on to the right leg. Left hand has come up in front of the right side of the body until it is in front of the right shoulder (palm facing inwards), elbow hanging down. The right hand has fallen (palm down) from outside the right shoulder to in front of the right hip. Gaze has just left the right hand and is about to be fixed on the left **completing** hand.   **an exhalation**

2. The small of the back turns a little to the left, weight moves slowly on to the left leg (for a split second a horse stance is struck as weight is being shifted from one leg to the other). The left hand (palm facing inwards) moves to the left with the turning of the small of the back, past the face until it is outside the left shoulder. The right hand (palm down) arcs to the left across the lower body in close harmony with the left hand until it is in front of the left hip.   **inhale**

3. With weight wholly on the left leg, the right foot steps to the left, coming to rest about 10-20 cm to the right of the left foot. The left hand turns palm down as it falls down to in front of the left hip. The right hand turns palm in as it pulls up to in front of the left shoulder, thumb pointing up.   **exhale**

4. The small of the back turns a little to the right, weight moves slowly on to the right leg. The right hand (palm facing inwards) moves to the right with the turning of the small of the back, past the face until it is outside the right shoulder. The left hand (palm down) arcs to the right across the lower body in close harmony

inhale with the right hand until it is in front of the right hip.

5. With weight wholly on the right leg, the left foot steps to the left sideways. The right hand turns palm down as it falls down to in front of the right hip. The left hand turns palm in as it pulls **exhale** up to in front of the right shoulder, thumb pointing up.

As can be seen from these examples, the basic principle here is the natural flow of close/hoard/inhale—open/release/exhale. This can be extended by analogy to all t'ai chi movements, thus enabling you to gradually harmonise breathing with every posture.

The key to knowing when to inhale and when to exhale is to think about the movements in terms of whether they are defensive or attacking martial arts movements. This is a matter of the experience which comes from continual practice and close analysis of the movements.

If you feel constriction in the chest or shortness of breath during the process of joining breathing and movements together, there must be something incorrect with your stance; and if the breathing doesn't fit evenly together with the movements, you must make adjustments. Very often all that is needed to bring breathing and movements together in their natural flow is a small adjustment to the tempo at which various movements or parts thereof are performed. If you are still feeling uncomfortable after adjusting the timing, you should revert to natural breathing rather than force the issue.

Each of the many styles of t'ai chi currently in vogue in both the East and the West has developed its own characteristics and peculiarities through long years of constant use and thoughtful study. But despite these variations and idiosyncracies, they all, without exception, adhere to the principle that the integration of consciousness, breathing and movements is primary.

This means that breathing and movements are to be coordinated by the conscious will, by consciousness. It is this conscious coordination that is responsible for promoting stronger and more healthy functioning of the internal organs.

At the heart of all the movements of all styles of t'ai chi is getting power moving in a spiral and, for this to happen, again it is essential that consciousness be coordinated with breathing and movements. When power moves in a spiral, and only then, is it possible to aspire to that level of expertise where *in moving, there is no place that does not move, there is no place power does not reach* and you are able to *lure an opponent into failure.*

Below is a table of correspondences used in the various styles of t'ai chi:

Inhale	Exhale
Close	Open
Hollow	Concrete
Hoard	Release
Bow down*	Stretch
Retreat	Advance
Rise	Fall
Look up*	Look down*
Come	Go
Enter	Leave
Gather in	Let go
Change	Strike
Lure	Attack
Soft	Hard
Yin	Yang

You will notice that the first four are inhale = closed = hollow = hoarding, and exhale = open = concrete = releasing. In the Ch'en, the Yang, both Wu and the Sun styles, each and every movement abides by this natural alternation between closed/open, hollow/concrete and inhale/exhale.

Open/closed = concrete/hollow = exhale/inhale has been laid down quite strictly for the movements of t'ai chi. It must be stressed, however, that only when this is a *natural coordination* between movements and breathing, and not a straitjacket rigidly conformed to, will *ch'i heal rather than impair*. Breathing deeply, slowly, thoroughly, evenly and easily is the most important injunction with regard to t'ai chi breathing.

*Note Bending the trunk forward or backward, and leaning to the left or right are considered to be faults in t'ai chi since, by doing any of these, the body loses its uprightness and sense of being comfortable; also, changes lack agility. The looking up and down and moving to either side mentioned here should not be misinterpreted as the trunk itself bending: what is meant is the moving up or down of inner power.

The statement in the Classic that *If he looks up then I go even higher, if he looks down then I go even lower* means that when an opponent approaches with his head up, I rise up so as to lure him, making him feel as though he is confronted by an unassailable towering weightlessness; and when an opponent approaches with his head down, I go down so as to lure him, making him feel as though he is tottering on the edge of an abyss which he is being sucked down into.

The Classic has it—*Move ch'i with the consciousness, making sure it is deep:* here *deep* means increasing the intensity of breathing. The Classic also says—*Move the body with ch'i, making sure it is smooth:* here *smooth* means increasing the volume of air in the lungs. These things should happen spontaneously and not be forced.

8. Open/Closed and Concrete/Hollow

In both the theory and the practice of t'ai chi ch'üan the concepts of open/closed and of concrete/hollow are of primary importance.

Open/closed is initiated from within, appears externally and is a matter of postures. Concrete/hollow is a matter of the heaviness or lightness of inner power. Breathing is a matter of the physiology of movement. The close and natural coordination of these three is what constitutes the unity of internal/external and the wholeness of the way in which t'ai chi trains mind, trains *ch'i* and trains body.

Some quotes from the T'ai Chi Classic about open/closed and concrete/hollow:

Open/closed and concrete/hollow are the warp of t'ai chi ch'üan;

In the alternation between open and closed there is change, there is constancy; concrete and hollow co-exist, suddenly appearing and suddenly disappearing;

There is closure in the midst of open and open in the midst of closure; there is hollow in the midst of concrete and concrete in the midst of hollow;

The subtlety of the art of t'ai chi ch'üan is completely embodied in the alternation between open and closed.

The moves from closed to open and from open to closed, as well as the transformations back and forth between concrete and hollow, are always gradual, never sudden. These moves and transformations fit in spatially with the startings and endings of the physical movements and take place temporally according to the tempo of their changes and motions. It is this leisurely and even style of movement that is particularly effective in the treatment and prevention of illness.

T'ai chi has always been a martial art of inner power. This means that movements and breathing must be linked together by the conscious exercise of the will. It also means that the intimate linking together of consciousness, breathing and movements allows the mind, the *ch'i* and the body to be trained simultaneously.

In this context, 'movements' includes the internal action of the muscles, the joints and the organs as well as the external actions of the trunk and the limbs. Internal and external movements can only become as one when internal action leads external form and external form coincides with internal action.

Open/Closed

1. Open/closed is the internal leading the external and the external guiding the internal.

Open/closed in t'ai chi is the integration of the internal with the external: the internal leads the external and the external guides the internal. Open and closed should spring from the internal and then become manifest externally.

Chinese masters have always laid particular stress on exercising the body's internal organs. It is held, therefore, that open/closed which merely takes on an external form without springing from an internal source diminishes its usefulness in therapy, in body-building and in martial arts skill. T'ai chi performed in this way must lack the quality of unity.

Open and closed are internal changes, they are not just a shape or appearance. However, as far as external shape is concerned, the movements of t'ai chi take the form of stretching/withdrawing, advancing/retreating, inclining forward/leaning backwards, falling/rising, etc.

When combined properly with breathing, the following external shapes are *open:* stretching, advancing, inclining forward, falling, etc.

Again when they are combined properly with breathing, the following external shapes are *closed:* withdrawing, retreating, leaning backwards, rising, etc.

The function of open/closed which springs from the internal is to get power moving in a spiral. This is what is meant by *power transforms from within* and *internal ch'i is transferred subtly.* Open is extending and enlarging; closed is contracting and restraining. The spiralling type of movements in t'ai chi have an adhesive quality: withdrawing is followed immediately by stretching, so that in being open there is no risk of extending yourself beyond your capacity and in being closed there is no sense of dodging away.

As you work on integrating open/closed internally and externally, it is useful to keep in mind the concept that if there is no movement within there can be no releasing externally.

With each and every movement consciousness initiates action, the internal continues the motion, which then becomes external movement. What you are aiming for is that as soon as movement is commenced, the internal and the external move together and form and spirit become as one.

2. There is closure in the midst of open and open in the midst of closure.

During open movements, both the internal and the external are completely open and during closed movements both the internal and the external are quite closed. The body is thus an entity which changes from one to the other at one and the same instant. This makes it possible for strength and power which are concentrated in a single point to be transferred agilely at will and be concentrated in any other point.

However, the essence of getting power moving in a spiral is that there be closure in the midst of open and open in the midst of closure. So, while open and closed alternate, there is yet a further step, and that is to have closure in the midst of open and open in the midst of closure.

Don't allow open to be simply open, and closed to be simply closed. In open there should be a sense of closed and hoarding; in closed a sense of open and releasing. It is only possible to support force from every direction and to change around to any direction when something is always held in reserve, when there is a surplus, when everything is strung together in one piece and both movement and stillness spring from a common source.

There is yet one further injunction. As well as there being closed in the midst of open and open in the midst of closed, *there is open in the midst of open, and the closed can be further closed. Open in the midst of open* is the capacity to extend spiral power even further as it goes forward; *the closed can be further closed* is the capacity to retract spiral power even further as it retreats.

Power which moves from the spine at the small of the back in a spiralling, arc-shaped fashion out towards the extremities of the limbs is called *open*. That which moves back in from the extremities to the *tan t'ien* is called *closed*.

Great emphasis is placed in t'ai chi on integrating internal and external movement. As you become more experienced, you should keep in mind the concept that if there is no movement within, there can be no releasing externally. The quintessence of the practice of t'ai chi is this acting from the inside out, which springs entirely from the spiralling of power.

Concrete/Hollow

Concrete/hollow is a matter of where consciousness or attention is focused. In the hands, for instance, concrete and hollow are differentiated as follows: if your mind focuses on the right hand then the right hand is concrete and the left hollow; if you focus on the left hand then it is concrete and the right hollow.

There is hollow in the midst of concrete and concrete in the midst of hollow.

Nevertheless, it is still necessary that there be hollow amidst the concrete and concrete amidst the hollow, so that in each of the respectively concrete or hollow hands described above there is yet a hint of hollow or concrete, as the case may be.

Hollow in the midst of concrete can again be exemplified by the hand. With a concrete hand that is pushing forward, the front or palm side is concrete while the back of that hand is hollow. This ensures that every other part of the body is not drained of strength in order to focus strength in a single point.

Nor should the hollow hand to the rear be ignored; if it is, it will lack taut strength. This having concrete amidst the hollow balances the body's centre of gravity as well as lending more power to the hand in front.

Every movement in t'ai chi involves circles and the transformation between concrete and hollow takes place within this circularity. While transforming alternately between concrete and hollow, however, there should still be a sense of power seeming to be relaxed yet not being relaxed, of hovering on the brink of unfolding, as you work gradually towards having hollow amidst the concrete and concrete amidst the hollow.

In the legs there is, of course, also transformation between concrete and hollow. Here again, there should be a gradual progression towards having hollow amidst the concrete and concrete amidst the hollow. This applies to the legs at all times, whether it is the front leg that is hollow and the rear concrete or vice versa, or whether it is the left leg that is hollow and the right concrete or vice versa. Work also towards ensuring that the concrete leg is not completely fixed and stagnant nor the hollow leg entirely without strength.

In the early stages of practising t'ai chi only concern yourself with differentiating between that leg which is concrete and that which is hollow. The leg in flight is hollow while the leg on which the body's weight falls is concrete; with concrete/hollow steps, the upper inner thighs should be held apart with the knees always slightly bent.

As you progress and gradually refine your movements, however, the ratio between concrete and hollow in the legs should diminish. That is to say, initially the ratio should be concrete : hollow 8 : 2. This ratio should diminish by degrees to concrete : hollow 7 : 3, then to concrete : hollow 6 : 4 and then to concrete : hollow 5.5 : 4.5, for the closer the ratio between concrete and hollow, the nimbler and quicker will transformations be able to be made.

The terms *yin* and *yang* have long been used interchangeably with closed and open and hollow and concrete. Closed and hollow are *yin:* open and concrete are *yang.* Thus, *there is yin in the midst of yang and yang in the midst of yin; there is closure in the midst of open and open in the midst of closure; and there is hollow in the midst of concrete and concrete in the midst of hollow* all mean one and the same thing.

Yin and yang, each of them is the source means that hollow and concrete should each permeate the other and imperceptibly influence the other. As well as permeating each other, concrete and hollow should suddenly appear and suddenly disappear, the transformations between them being exceptionally deft.

Concrete and hollow can suddenly appear and suddenly disappear only when there is deft transformation between consciousness and *ch'i*. And this nimble transformation between consciousness and *ch'i* operates on the internal/external and the upper/lower links as well as in the legs, as does the sense of liveliness thus achieved.

Like the moves between open and closed, the transformations between concrete and hollow are initiated from within by consciousness and are reflected in external movements, so that internal and external become as one.

Every movement and posture in t'ai chi involves open/closed and concrete/hollow transforming alternately between each other with the flow and change of movement. If the mind is required to concentrate continuously on a single hand or if it must concentrate on both hands as they travel together in the same direction, then it is the open/closed of the movement which dictates the transformation between concrete and hollow. In other words, a movement which is open will be concrete and a movement which is closed will be hollow.

Breathing

The harmony between the movements of the internal and the external is characterised by withdrawing/stretching, closed/open, and the transformation between hollow and concrete. Permeating the movements of t'ai chi is its distinctive and unique way of getting power moving in a spiral. When internal movements harmonise with external movements, breathing must be combined naturally and rhythmically with both.

If you get out of step or don't concentrate on the natural coordination of closed = hollow and open = concrete with your breathing, and arbitrarily insert an additional movement that demands either an inhalation or an exhalation, then of course that movement cannot flow into the natural coordination already established between breathing and movements. To compensate for the interruption, therefore, you will have to take a short breath or expel a little air. But both breathing and movements should then revert to their natural coordination.

Closed and hollow are hoarding. Open and concrete are releasing. There should be an easy and natural coordination between breathing and the actions of open/closed and concrete/

hollow. To open and then to close is to exhale and then inhale. One exhalation and one inhalation is counted as a complete breath.

Concrete and hollow should not be understood as merely distinguishing between concrete and hollow in the hands and the feet. There should, in fact, be a clear differentiation between concrete and hollow in the muscles, the bones and the functioning of the organs of the chest, the abdomen and the back. This, really, is the major differentiation in the movements, for if concrete and hollow are distinguished between only in the hands and feet and not in the chest, the abdomen and the back, then the internal is not controlling the external.

To see just the limbs working in concert with the internal action of a complete breath as being the martial art of inner power is to see only part of the picture. Merely breathing so that the diaphragm moves up and down, and believing that this will initiate gentle massage of the internal organs, is to discount the role of consciousness in guiding into movement the muscles, the bones and the functioning of the organs of the chest, the abdomen and the back. Only an entwining style of circular movement can stimulate the internal organs, the muscles, the blood, the main and collateral channels and the spinal cord into motion. Such a style of circular movement gets power moving in a spiral and moves *ch'i* as though through a pearl with nine passages, so that there's not the tiniest space it doesn't penetrate.

Closed and hollow are inhalations. So with closing movements such as bowing down, retreating, leaning backwards and commencing, you should inhale. While gradually transforming from concrete to hollow you should also inhale.

Open and concrete are exhalations. So with opening movements such as stretching, advancing, inclining forward and completing, you should exhale. While gradually transforming from hollow to concrete you should also exhale.

After many years of practice, adepts enjoy a freedom of transformation in that they are able to move rapidly and make abrupt transformations between open and closed and concrete and hollow. In general, however, lightning fast movements are only advocated for purposes of attack and defence. *In a crisis respond with rapidity, otherwise move slowly.*

Here is a specific example of the close coordination between breathing and the internal/external integration of open/closed and concrete/hollow. The movement is *As Though Sealing Up* which follows (Revolving) Block Punch.

In the first part of this movement, as the body slowly sits back and the right fist changes back to an open hand, both hands separate away from each other and pull back in to the chest, palms tilting slightly inwards. The external form of this movement is that of closing, bowing down and retreating. In terms of concrete/hollow, it is a gradual transformation from concrete to hollow. This movement calls for an inhalation. As you inhale, the diaphragm rises and the abdomen pulls in a little as the muscles in the chest move up, the chest cavity relaxes out and the power of the crotch sinks downwards: this is hoarding.

In the second part of this movement the hands press forward, palms turning forward. This is an opening, stretching and advancing movement and is a gradual transformation from hollow to concrete. This movement calls for an exhalation. As you exhale, the diaphragm falls and the abdomen pushes out a little (ch'i sinks to the tan t'ien) while the muscles in the chest sink in a curving motion down the sides to skirt the abdomen and come together at the centre of the body in front of the abdomen. The muscles moving in this way unify strength immensely and allow a forward release of power: this is releasing power.

This is how closed/open, hollow/concrete, hoarding/releasing, inhaling/exhaling operates. The first movement is closed, hollow, hoarding, inhaling. The second part is open, concrete, releasing, exhaling.

The way in which *power transforms from within* is also an alternation between the large and small muscles of the chest and a changing in the small of the back. Alternation in the chest is what happens when the muscles of the chest fluctuate as they curve up and down, right and left in conjunction with the body's external movements. Changing in the small of the back is what happens when, as the lower limbs change between concrete and hollow, the kidney on the same side as the concrete foot assumes a sense of concreteness, seeming to compensate for the other kidney on the same side as the hollow foot. The T'ai Chi Classic refers to this latter phenomenon when it says: *The source of life and consciousness lies in the crevices of the small of the back (the kidneys); Deeply involve the consciousness in the region of the small of the back;* and *In advancing and retreating there must be transformation.*

There is a unity in the alternations evident externally in the hands and those in the legs, and each of them involves both the internal and the external. Thus to explain this alternation and change merely in terms of what the hands and feet can be seen to be doing is, again, only a partial explanation which ignores control of the external by the internal and lacks internal/external unity.

Taut strength cannot possibly be lost if bowing down and retreating movements are always arc-shaped and coiling. But if they are not, then taut strength will become feeble weakness which is merely hollow, lacking concrete in the midst of hollow. Inner power which seems to be relaxed, but is not relaxed, is the magic that results from there being concrete in the midst of hollow.

With stretching and advancing movements, even if they appear to be following a straight line of travel, inner power flows forward in a spiral. Hollow in the midst of concrete is when inner power lingers and winds, neither soft nor hard, on the verge of unfurling without being direct or still. Exceptionally nimble transformations in which there is both an easy agility and a heaviness comes with long practice.

Inhaling on closed, hollow and hoarding; exhaling on open, concrete and releasing. These are completely natural physiological correspondences. Let us look again at the example just cited, *As Though Sealing Up*:

In the first part of this movement as the hands pull back in towards the chest, the limbs and trunk relax and withdraw while consciousness gradually moves from concrete to hollow. Because the body is slowly sitting back, the muscles, bones, etc. of the chest, ribs and back gently contract. This contraction makes the diaphragm contract as well so that the chest cavity is expanded: the lungs automatically inhale. This is open in the midst of closed because of the simultaneous contraction and expansion.

In the second part of the movement as both hands push forward, the process is reversed. Consciousness gradually moves from hollow to concrete and, because the body is slowly reaching forward, the muscles, bones, etc. of the chest, ribs, stomach and back gently stretch. This stretching allows the diaphragm to revert to its original convex shape so that the capacity of the chest cavity is reduced: the lungs automatically exhale. This is closed in the midst of open because both expansion and contraction are involved.

The T'ai Chi Classic points out that open and closed are not in fact definite, for bowing and stretching stances are linked together. Throughout t'ai chi, therefore, every movement should be coordinated rhythmically and naturally with breathing. Inhaling on closed and hollow, and exhaling on open and concrete is in no way forced or artificial since it corresponds quite naturally with the dictates of human physiology.

On exhaling with opening and releasing, the diaphragm descends. The pressure this exerts on the abdomen makes the abdomen expand and allows the body's centre of gravity to sink down, while pressure in the chest is lessened and it contracts.

On inhalation with closing and hoarding, the diaphragm ascends. This relieves pressure on the abdomen, which contracts, and causes the body's centre of gravity to move up higher, while the increased pressure in the chest makes it expand and increases the capacity of the lungs.

The tempo at which you breathe is dictated by the movements and postures, for pressure on the abdomen and on the chest alternates as you breathe and as the body moves from one posture to another. In this way the internal organs are stimulated and toned up and the circulation of blood and ch'i speeded up, while the power of hoarding and of release are heightened, and accurate adjustments in the body's centre of gravity become easier.

9. Symmetry and Accord

Coherence and roundedness in t'ai chi springs from the muscles being relaxed. And when the muscles of the whole body are consciously controlled, movements become precise, compact, structured, disciplined and unified. With such movements, instead of there being an imbalance caused by each of the joints pulling disparately in different directions, there is in every movement a focusing of strength. This is described as *symmetry and accord, or ch'i and stance reunited.*

That symmetry and accord wherein *ch'i* and stances do not lack unity can be achieved if at all times you seek to focus your strength. Essential to the coherence and roundedness of t'ai chi is an intrinsic symmetry and accord, for without this intrinsic symmetry and accord there will be only external form lacking in substance.

There are five aspects to this intrinsic symmetry and accord and in this chapter a practical example is given of how each of these principles is applied. These are fairly complex concepts but they are worth pondering, for their delight lies in their very complexity.

1. The intention of ascending implies first descending.
The instant of closure, hollow and hoarding has just been

reached when both hands have pulled back in to the body, weight has shifted on to the back leg and an inhalation is just being completed.

Then, with the change in direction to press or push forward, the ribs are first drawn down in an arc by the muscles on both sides of the chest. At the same time an exhalation begins, with some of the air being expelled and some sinking down. The hips pull in a fraction and sink down, shoulders are heavy, elbows hanging and the hands also sink fractionally down in an arc.

Moving along with the forward motion of the small of the back and the legs, the inner power of both sides of the abdomen immediately changes direction to arc forward and up in exactly the same direction as the shallow arcing up and pushing forward of the hands, so that strength focuses in a single point. The power of the crotch sinks down and then rises up a little as the halfway point of the body's travel is reached (this must not be an obvious bobbing up and down, but is rather an internal process).

Throughout, the body should be upright, with no hollows, humps, discontinuities or leaning to either side, and the movements should be calm and rounded without any rigidity. This is open, concrete and releasing power.

2. Intending to go to the left, you must first go to the right.

When about to step out with the left leg, the right kidney first rotates down, the right hip rotates to the right and pulls inwards and weight moves on to the right leg. Then the left knee lifts up, the left hip opens out and the left foot slowly reaches out until the heel lightly touches the ground. When stepping out to the right the converse applies.

Whether turning to the left or to the right, the body should be kept erect, with all movements in harmony. Be careful that the shoulders remain level and do not drop out of their proper horizontal alignment with each other.

3. In the midst of going forward, there must be an anchoring back.

As the body, the hands and the legs move forward, the power of the crotch sinks down and there is strength in the soles of the feet. Inner power rolls from the crotch up along the spine, penetrates to the fingers and shoots directly ahead. But the *ming men point** anchors backwards. The hands push forward,

*Note: The *ming men* point is between the second and the third vertebrae of the small of the back.

extending power, but there is a sense of pulling back inwards in the backs of the hands.

This is the symmetry and accord of *where there is in front, there must be behind.* It may also be described as stretching from both in front and behind, the aim being to secure the body's centred, comfortable bearing and give greater kick-back or reflex strength.

4. *Upper/lower and left/right are intimately related.*

The left leg steps lightly out in front, angled towards the left, and the right arm gently extends back, angled towards the right. The fingers of the right hand come to rest diagonally over the toes of the right foot and the left arm follows closely as it, too, moves to the right and comes to rest in front of the right shoulder.

There should be a sense of echoing and interrelationship upper/lower and left/right between the toes of both feet, between the fingers of both hands, and between the fingers and the toes of both hands and feet. This imparts to the movement an air of unfolding which does not lack unity, a feeling that the spirit is still whole and that, in unfolding, what is in reserve has not drained away. This, in fact, is what is meant by there being closure in the midst of open.

It is primarily because of the support provided by the static concrete right leg that the dynamic hollow left leg which is stepping out is able to move nimbly forward; but unless the right side of the chest also feels related to the left leg, the hollow left leg will tend towards flightiness.

5. *Stretch from both ends and in the curved seek the straight.*

This fifth principle of stretching from both ends and seeking the straight amidst the curved is one which permeates t'ai chi in its every aspect.

(a) In stretching from above and below, seek the straight amidst the curved:

The vertebrae are relaxed down and sitting vertical, and the tailbone is full of strength. *Ch'i* has sunk to the *tan t'ien*, the power of the crotch has sunk down and the power of the soles of the feet seems to be thrusting into the ground like the roots of a tree. Yet the whole time, the *pai hui* point guides delicately upwards. This is the technique of suspended crown, *ch'i* sinking to the *tan t'ien* and lifting head, suspended crotch which stretches from above and below.

At the same time, in the upper torso, the chest is held and the back drawn, with the large vertebra at the top of the back pulling upwards. In the lower torso, the lower abdomen is thrusting forward, with the *ming men* point on the spine at the small of the back anchoring backwards. Each of the spinal vertebrae is relaxed down and delicately resting on the one below so that the whole spinal column is flexible yet providing firm support. In this easy stance of the trunk, the trunk is erect and the spinal column retains its natural curvature.

(b) Hands and feet stretch from both ends, seeking the straight amidst the curved:

Knees are bent, the soles of the feet treading firmly as if their power were thrusting into the ground like the roots of a tree. Yet their power also lifts upwards in the heels, giving the feet a sense of springing against the ground. The hands stretch forward, extending power, yet the shoulders still relax down and the elbows still hang down bent, not straight, to lend a heavier power to the arms. The power of the feet is treading down, the power of the hands releasing out forward.

(c) Stretching from both ends during entwining movement:

Still echoing each other, the hands are moving away from each other, either one to the left and the other to the right, or one up and the other down. The hip joints are held open and each of the knees thrusts forward in a different direction from the other.

PART 4
BECOMING AN ADEPT

10. T'ai Chi Techniques

Introduction

So that they can be most easily grasped and digested, the t'ai chi techniques which are explained here are presented in sections as they relate to each part of the body.

Although these techniques are segmented according to the parts of the body, it should always be remembered that the physical body is an entity composed of interrelated and interdependent parts. The techniques themselves, therefore, should be thought of as being relevant to the whole body and not compartmentalised as being specifically relevant to one part of the body only and not to any other. Retain always an overall perspective in your gradual mastery of the techniques so that each helps rather than hinders the others.

One by one incorporate them into your practice so that a solid foundation is laid down in the proper ways of using your arms, legs, body and eyes. By practising them over and over again from the very beginning you will gradually be able to make them an integral part of t'ai chi postures. And once in control of the tempo, direction and intricacies of the actual movements, you can continue the gradual process of becoming an adept by consistent practice. Little by little your stance will improve, your movements will round out, upper and lower will interact and your whole body will begin to work in harmony.

After you have become familiar with the basic outline of the movements of whichever style of t'ai chi you are learning, concentrate in the quiet of your own mind on only one technique at a time. Move through them one by one at your own pace until you feel you are beginning to understand both intellectually and physically what is being asked of you by them.

It is not intended that you should necessarily start with the head and work systematically down through the body. It would be best to choose the technique which appeals most to you or which you feel to be the easiest and work on that one first. Then go on to another which you feel to be both important and comfortable.

Some of them will probably seem rather abstruse or even downright unintelligible to begin with. But as you continue to practise t'ai chi thoughtfully and consistently, you will in time gain insight into the more difficult and abstract concepts involved.

For ease of reference and of use, these techniques can be summarised broadly as twelve maxims:

1. Quiet heart, relaxed body
2. Centred, at ease
3. Suspended crown
4. *Ch'i* sinking to the *tan t'ien*
5. Hold the chest, draw the back
6. Heavy shoulders, hanging elbows
7. Seated wrists, open palms
8. Relaxed small of the back, restrained buttocks
9. Tailbone at dead centre
10. Bent knees, relaxed hips
11. Differentiation between concrete and hollow in the legs
12. Upper and lower on a single cord

These techniques do not come easily and you will need to be persistent in your efforts to incorporate them. But always remember that blind, mechanical practice of t'ai chi is of very little value. Always practise t'ai chi thoughtfully. Be aware of what you are doing and what you are aiming for. With consistent practice you will then be able to pick up and correct all deviations from what is held to be the most effective use of your body in t'ai chi.

A. Head and Neck

1. Head

Hold the head erect the whole time you are doing t'ai chi. If the head and neck are held upright, the trunk will respond by straightening up into a naturally upright posture. Standing straight and tall and looking the world right in the eye is synonymous with vitality and vigour, while hunched shoulders, a stoop and a drooping head are symbolic of old age and decrepitude. A hunched-over stoop need not develop with advancing age, however, and consistent, regular practice of t'ai chi will soon be reflected in the way you hold yourself.

Holding the head erect simply means consciously preventing the head dropping forward, bending backward or tilting over to either side. Whether in a stance or in flight, imagine there is a light and extremely valuable object resting on the very top of the head, and then you will not be able to drop your head down, tip it back or let it fall aslant.

When the body turns, the head should be kept level and steady so that it doesn't wag about or tip over to one side.

It is very tempting when you start learning t'ai chi to assume a special fey 'I'm doing t'ai chi' look, but it is important that from the start the facial muscles be allowed to relax into their normal expression.

In a posture, look straight ahead of the body and fix your gaze on some distant point. In flight, your gaze should follow the movement of the leading hand or foot. Your gaze should have a definite focus, but at the same time you should be visually aware of your surroundings and not stare fixedly off into space.

Gaze moves with the hands, while vision is all-encompassing. This dictum derives from t'ai chi's status as a sibling in the martial arts family, but its practical function is that by continually changing the focus of the gaze from a distant object to a near one the optical nerves are being given exercise as well. Over a period of time you can expect from this an improvement in your sight: vision will be sharpened and that sparkle will return to your eye.

With the tongue lifting slightly to the palate, hold the lips and teeth lightly together. The resultant increase in the flow of saliva will stop the throat becoming dry and will aid the digestive process.

Always breathe through the nose. Breathe naturally, aiming gradually to coordinate breathing and movements. If at any stage you feel breathless, take a short breath through the mouth to relieve the discomfort. The key is to breathe unhurriedly and naturally.

So that it doesn't jut out awkwardly, the chin should be drawn in just a little. Don't pull it in too far, though, or breathing will be hampered and the attitudes of suspended crown and drawn back will both suffer.

Aurally, be aware of the sounds behind and around you. A spirit at ease and a body at peace sharpens the sense of hearing.

2. Crown of the Head

Special emphasis is given in t'ai chi to what is known as suspended crown. Suspended crown is a very, very delicate guiding upwards with the power of the crown of the head.

Located on the top of the skull towards the back of the head (directly over the tops of the ears) is an acupuncture point called the *pai hui* point, and the power of the crown of the head derives from the *pai hui* point lifting very lightly upwards as though it were suspended by a cord.

As with all these t'ai chi techniques, suspended crown does not operate in isolation. Beneath the trunk, just forward of the anus, is located another acupuncture point called the *hui yin* point. The special relevance of the *hui yin* point to suspended crown is that the head and trunk should be held in such a way that the *hui yin* and the *pai hui* points are always in a direct straight line with each other. The dictum that upper and lower be on a single cord is just this attitude of keeping the *pai hui* point and the *hui yin* point in the one perpendicular line.

Suspended crown helps both form and function in the following ways:

(a) Suspended crown helps keep the head erect because of the tautness of the imaginary cord suspending the crown of the head which will not allow the head to loll forward, backward or sideways.

(b) By causing the spinal column to stretch along its entire length, suspended crown facilitates the regulatory tasks of the central nervous system. And by bringing the body into proper alignment, it allows the body's balance mechanism to operate more naturally.

(c) The skull being suspended by a cord lends to the body a

feeling of lightness and a lessening of pressure down upon it; this brings with it an appearance of agility in the way the body moves.

(d) There is a very intimate relationship between suspended crown and *ch'i* sinking to the *tan t'ien*. Suspended crown lifts the spirit while *ch'i* sinking to the *tan t'ien* stabilises the body's centre of gravity. From this upper/lower symmetry springs a taut power which seems to be relaxed yet is not relaxed, a taut power brimming with elasticity and pliability. A surging up of vigour also stems from this symmetry, since it impels a natural lifting of the spirit, increases excitation of the nerves and relaxes open the entire body.

The *pai hui* point should reach up neither too much nor too little; there must be no hint of straining upwards, but a very delicate, intangible guiding upwards. In the same way, *ch'i* sinking to the *tan t'ien* must not be a squashing heavily downwards of the *ch'i* but an intangible pouring of consciousness into the *tan t'ien*. Consciousness held in the *tan t'ien* is resting power, having the sense of keeping the abdomen static; consciousness pouring into the *tan t'ien* is mobile power which, concentrated on the abdomen, has a dynamic sense. Mastering suspended crown and *ch'i* sinking to the *tan t'ien* lends to all the movements of t'ai chi a light agility, a wholeness, a steadiness and a firmness.

(e) The *pai hui* point maintaining an attitude of suspended crown gives the entire body a focal point. Also, the lower jaw automatically retracts a little when the attitude of suspended crown is assumed and this is extremely important with relation to both even breathing and the imperceptible inner shifts in vital energy.

But if the front of the skull is held higher than the *pai hui* point, the chin will be forced too far forward and if the rear of the skull is held higher than the *pai hui* point, the chin will be forced too far in towards the throat. Aim, therefore, to achieve a nice balance between the *pai hui* point guiding up very delicately, the lower jaw drawing in easily and *ch'i* nestling against the spine.

3. Neck

Held quite upright and relaxed, the neck should be neither rigid nor limp. If the neck is rigid and stiff, or over-relaxed to the extent of becoming limp, turning movements around to the sides will be directly affected in that they will lack ease and agility. As well as this, it will be impossible to hold the head in an attitude of suspended crown, and the strain of holding the neck rigid will be reflected in a tightening of the muscles of the face.

The extent to which the crown is suspended is a crucial factor in holding the neck upright and relaxed: if the *pai hui* point guides up excessively the neck will become rigid, but if it does not guide up sufficiently the result will be a limp, flaccid neck.

At the very base of the skull between the two tendons running up the back of the neck is located the *ya men* acupuncture point. At the very base of the spine just below the coccyx is located another acupuncture point called the *ch'ang ch'iang* point. These two acupuncture points move in harmony with each other. The *ya men* point is on the first cervical vertebra which is capable of movement and when this vertebra rotates the skull acts as a pivot maintaining balance and centring the head.

Suspended crown is what maintains the head and the spinal column in the correct state of equilibrium. The resiliency of the spinal column has earned it the nickname in t'ai chi of 'the living bow'. In one of the Wu styles the grip of this bow is the small of the back, while the tips of the bow are, respectively, the large vertebra at the top of the back and the tailbone at the base of the spine. In the Ch'en style the upper tip of the bow is taken to be the *ya men* point on the topmost cervical vertebra, because extending it upwards to that point increases the bow's degree of regulation and of explosive strength. Just as suspended crown acts as a balance for the spinal column, so the cervical vertebrae act as modulators.

When practising t'ai chi, the neck moves in the same direction as the eyes.

B. Upper Limbs

1. Shoulders

In t'ai chi, sometimes the body leads the hands and sometimes the hands lead the body, but this does not alter the fact that movements of the upper limbs always flow with the postures and revolve, encircle. The hands and arms, therefore, need to be relaxed and lively while they are stretching out, pulling back, revolving and encircling.

The ability of the hands and arms to be relaxed and nimble, however, depends entirely on the shoulder joints being able to open out. This opening out of the shoulder joints is a conscious process which takes time to achieve, but once the movements have been learned thoroughly, the shoulder joints will of themselves gradually open out and sink downwards.

Shoulders must be heavy before they can relax, then once the shoulder joints are relaxed down completely the stretching, withdrawing and entwining of the hands and arms will have the grace of a windblown willow and a liveliness completely devoid of the mechanical.

One of the most important injunctions of t'ai chi is to have heavy shoulders and hanging elbows. Heavy shoulders and hanging elbows help in holding the chest and drawing the back, while lifted shoulders and elbows that poke out detract from it and adversely affect ch'i sinking to the tan t'ien.

This is what 'holding the chest' means: with the collarbone relatively stable, yet slightly sunk, the chest muscles relax and the chest cavity, held slightly in without being either concave or convex, feels relaxed inside.

This is what 'drawing the back' means: the back muscles relax, shoulder blades spread out and feel heavy so that the arms hang by the sides with enough space for a fist to fit under the armpit. The back muscles pull on the vertebrae so that they sit vertically, directly on top of one another, with the large vertebra between the shoulder joints seeming to be pulling the spinal column upwards and making the skin in that area feel taut.

As an aid to holding the chest and drawing the back, both the Ch'en and one of the Wu styles of t'ai chi advocate that the shoulders also curl very slightly forward. This slight curling forward of the shoulders promotes both taut power and focused strength, especially when it is associated with an arc-shaped relaxing down of the rib cage and the muscles around the rib cage, a compact abdomen and a pulling forward of the muscles running down the sides of the chest.

If the shoulders are relaxed and heavy and rotate freely, the ligaments and muscles in the shoulder region will be able to stretch and this stretching will form the back muscles into the proper shape to allow ch'i to nestle against the spine.

When you begin to learn t'ai chi you need think only of relaxing the whole body; think of the shoulders, too, from the point of view of relaxing.

As you improve technique and begin to understand the transformations between concrete and hollow, you should think in terms of sinking down. Think specifically of the shoulders in terms of sinking down, allowing inner power to sink down rather than merely be soft, and the hands and arms to be extremely light and lively yet also extremely lithe and heavy. In this way the hands and arms will gradually grow in the elastic and pliant taut power that seems to pause yet does not pause, and has hardness and softness coexisting within it.

With heavy shoulders and hanging elbows take care that there is enough room under the armpits to put a fist. Arms must not hug the ribs, elbows should be away from the ribs so that the hands and arms have ample room to manoeuvre. This also ensures that the elasticity and pliability inherent in opening out power and not allowing it to be bent is not lost.

Shoulders should be kept level. Avoid raising one and lowering the other when turning the body, as this spoils the appearence of having an upright body.

In every posture shoulders and hips should rest on the one vertical line. With the shoulders relaxed, heavy and curling very slightly forward and with a suggestion of holding the chest and drawing the back, it is as though the shoulder joints were threaded through by a cord, so that each moves in harmony with the other. This brings with it a sense of gathering together in the midst of stretching out, and this increases both taut power and focused strength.

In flight, whether advancing, retreating or turning to the left or right, a vertical line aligning upper and lower must be preserved between the shoulders and the hips so that upper and lower will be on a single cord.

2. Elbows

Elbows should always be slightly bent and possess power which seems to hang downwards. Even in *Crane's Wings*, for example, where the right hand and forearm are raised above shoulder level, the tip of the elbow should still possess power which hangs downwards.

An elbow which lifts up possesses lifting power, which is considered neither desirable nor useful power within t'ai chi. To allow the elbows to jut out away from the body hinders heavy shoulders and adversely affects ch'i sinking to the *tan t'ien*. Since it leaves the ribs quite exposed, jutting the elbows out also puts one at a serious disadvantage insofar as martial arts attack and defence are concerned.

Heavy shoulders and hanging elbows add strength to the hands and arms in their stretching, withdrawing and entangling, and are essential to properly sitting wrists.

Elbows should respond to the knees in every stance, and there should be a harmony between the elbows above and below, in front and behind, and to the left and the right.

3. Wrists

The wrists are capable of a very great degree of rotation and are the most flexible joints of the entire body. What you should work towards with regard to the wrists is the technique known as sitting wrists.

Many students, quite unaware of the importance of sitting wrists, seek only grace and nimbleness in the way they rotate their wrists in t'ai chi. It is extremely easy to allow the strength of the wrists to degenerate into weakness having a semblance of the nimble beauty that the graceful wrists of a dancer have, but lacking the strong beauty that comes from agility. This graceful weakness, however, makes it very difficult for inner power to penetrate to the very tips of the fingers and it adversely affects the accumulation of taut power in the hands and arms.

Wrists should be neither stiff nor weak, but should revolve pliably and flexibly as the hands and arms stretch out, withdraw and entangle.

'Sitting wrists' (also called settled wrists) is that technique whereby in a posture, along with the lowering of the hips, the settling of the small of the back, the sinking of ch'i and so on, the wrists also sink down and coax inner power very, very slowly into the palms. What sitting wrists does is allow the palms of the hands to control the flow of inner power so that it neither lingers overlong nor dissipates entirely.

4. Hands

The hands are the most dexterous part of the body and can assume many different shapes. In t'ai chi hand movements are differentiated into the palm, the fist and the hook, which shall each be dealt with separately.

(a) The Palm

The movements of the palm can be classified according to the direction and shape of the hand as follows:

Straight palm: fingertips pointing upwards, palm facing forward.

Upright palm: fingertips pointing or slanting upwards, palm facing in some other direction than forward.

F

Hanging palm: fingertips pointing or slanting downwards, palm facing in any direction.

Elevated palm: fingertips pointing in any direction, palm facing or slanting upwards.

Inclined palm: tip of the thumb pointing upwards, palm erect but on an angle and facing in any direction.

Lowered palm: fingertips pointing in any direction, palm facing or slanting downwards.

Reversed palm: thumb down, palm erect but on an angle.

The characteristic feature of the palm in t'ai chi is that the fingers are stretched out lightly, as opposed to the long-fist type of palm movement in the martial arts where the thumb is curled in tightly and the fingers are held straight and close together.

In the beginning the main point to watch is that when the palm is pushing forward and retracting, it is stretched out in a natural way. The fingers should neither be held tightly together nor be stretched rigidly out away from each other, and the palm of the hand should not be hollowed out.

When once you understand how movements are concrete and hollow, you should apply this concept to the palms as well as to the other parts of the body. Here is an example:

When the palm is about to push forward but has not yet started to move, it has a slightly hollow shape as if something were still held in reserve: this is a hollow palm.

As the palm pushes forward, curling and revolving, it gradually opens out and begins to lose the hollow: this is moving from hollow to concrete.

When the movement has been completed the hollow has all but disappeared, the fingers are slightly spread out, the wrist is sitting, and the heel of the hand is jutting forward a tiny bit so as to add to the forward stretch of the posture and to allow power to penetrate consciously to the tips of the fingers: this is a concrete palm.

As the palm withdraws, curling and revolving, it gradually reverts to seeming to hold something in reserve and starts to regain its slightly hollow shape: this is moving from concrete to hollow.

The movements of the palms of the hands are but one part of the movements of a whole, so concrete and hollow in the palm must be integrated with the changes between concrete and hollow of the whole. The integration of the movements of the hands with those of the small of the back, the legs and the feet is described thus in the T'ai Chi Classic: *originating in the feet, coming forth in the legs, controlled by the small of the back and assuming form in the fingers... all must be integrated and intact.*

You will eventually reach the stage in t'ai chi where you are able to activate every iota of *ch'i* and every vestige of power. When that happens, the alternation of power in the fingertips should, along with the stretching and entangling of the arms and forearms as they travel in different directions, progress to a variation between primary power and secondary power.

For example, when pushing forward with an inclined palm the tip of the little finger, which is in front, guides power forward, Then as the hand and forearm rotate forward, the focus of power moves from the tip of the little finger to the ring finger, to the middle finger, to the index finger and then on to the tip of the thumb so that inner power passes through the base of each of the five digits.

When it is the thumb that is guiding power forward, the focus of power moves through the fingers in turn along to the tip of the little finger as the hand and forearm rotate forward.

When raising or lowering a hand that is flat or level, the tip of the middle finger should guide power for, when power has penetrated quite through to that fingertip, the other digits of the hand will be filled with power as well.

Turning or twining the thumb outwards as the hand moves is called outward or flow turning; twining it inwards as the hand moves is called inward or counter turning. With both flow turning and counter turning it is very important that taut power is not lost from the hands. Taut power is that power which seems to be relaxed yet is not relaxed, that power in which hardness and softness coexist.

In the Ch'en and one of the Wu styles of t'ai chi the gaze rests on the tip of the middle finger, while in the Yang and the other Wu styles it rests on the tip of the index finger or on the thumb.

Whichever fingertip the eyes focus on when in a posture is taken to be the principal fingertip. Directed by consciousness, not by effort, inner power should penetrate very slowly through to the principal fingertip. Once power has penetrated quite through to the one fingertip, the other fingers will be full of power as well. The next posture can be initiated, then, as soon as power has penetrated quite through.

The spiralling, entangling movements of the hands and arms in t'ai chi is what makes it possible for power to travel across from finger to finger in the way described above. If the hands are brought straight up or lowered on a straight vertical path, this means of using and transmitting power will be quite unattainable.

In every stance the tips of the fingers and the tips of the toes should echo to each other above and below, or in front and behind as the case may be, just as the fingertips of each hand should echo to those of the other hand.

In most postures the fingertips should be level with and in line with the tip of the nose. In the vast majority of postures the tips of the fingers, the tips of the toes and the tip of the nose should line up with each other. Martial artists describe this apposition as *three tips in relation,* or *three tips in relation guarding the centre.*

Two last points. The first is that, so as not to disturb your balance, the palm of the hand should not descend beyond the knees when it presses downwards. The second is that the arms should never straighten completely but should retain at all times a slight curve which has a sense of holding something in reserve.

(b) The Fist

The fist in t'ai chi is formed in exactly the same way as in other martial arts. The four fingers are held together and, with the tip of the middle finger guiding, they are curled in until the fingertips are touching the palm of the hand; the ball of the thumb is then placed on the middle joint of the middle finger.

Although t'ai chi is that style of martial art wherein hardness dwells in softness, the starting point is always softness. The fist, therefore, should not be clenched too tightly, but there must still be an overall sense of coherence so that the fist can neither be prised open nor shattered under attack.

There are five attacking movements in t'ai chi that use the fist. These Five T'ai Chi Punches are:

concealing the hand and punching with the arm (Revolving Block Punch);
unleashing the body punch;
tip of the elbow punch;
striking the ground punch (Falling Punch);
punch towards the crotch.

Movements in t'ai chi consist of an interlacing of the straight and the reverse, looking down and looking up, the horizontal and the perpendicular, and this interlacing of opposites gives the movements their extremely varied outward form. The spiral and entangling motion characteristic of t'ai chi is very important in this regard, but care must be taken that the wrist has a relaxed strength and that the back of the hand doesn't buckle when it is driven downwards.

When the fist drives downwards, the back of the hand must be in a direct line with the armpit; it shouldn't trace a looping or curved path simply for the sake of appearance. The reason for this is the principle common to all the martial arts that unless the back of the hand drops down in a direct line from the armpit the wrist is very likely to suffer damage when resistance is encountered.

After a time you will realise that in the complex stretching, withdrawing and revolving of the fist, the focus of power in it alters.

For example, when stretching forward with an upright fist (the space between the thumb and index finger uppermost), the flat of the little finger between the back of the hand and the first joint guides power.

When striking forward with a level fist (palm facing downwards), the knuckle at the base of the middle finger guides it.

When the fist drives downwards, the first knuckle of the middle finger guides it.

When the fist punches upwards, the knuckle at the base of the middle finger guides it.

When the fist is circling either upwards (space between the thumb and index finger uppermost) or downwards (the bone at the outside of the wrist turning either in or out and the space between the thumb and index finger down), the knuckle of the thumb guides it.

When the fist chops down (space between the thumb and index finger uppermost), the knuckle at the base of the little finger guides it.

But when the bone at the outside of the wrist is turning out (with the space between the thumb and index finger slanting downwards), it is the knuckle at the base of the index finger which guides it.

Changes in the focus of power are dictated by the direction and purpose of the fist, the only criterion being that power be able to penetrate through to the fist.

(c) The Hook

The hook strengthens the wrist and the fingers and in the art of attack is used to capture: the hook is used to seize, to grasp, to ensnare and to capture.

Capturing movements in t'ai chi seek as their quarry membranes, veins, tendons and acupuncture points. To do this the hands are used in ways which restrain, grasp, clutch and obstruct because, since their target is sought through rubbing and pushing, they are not merely confined to countering muscle and bone.

In the Ch'en style there are several methods of capturing. Two ways of using the hands to capture in, for example, such transitional postures as covering the hand and punching with the forearm, are the hook where the four fingers curl in in a seizing motion, and the hook where the little and the ring fingers curl in and the index finger points straight ahead.

Usually deriving from a flat hand, i.e. not a fist, the hook is formed by gathering all five digits together so that the tips of the fingers either hang downwards or point towards the rear.

In t'ai chi there are two styles of hook.

With the hook in the Ch'en and one of the Wu styles, the little finger curls in first and then the ring, the middle and the index fingers in turn curl in. The tip of the little finger presses firmly against the heel of the hand and the thumb sits on the last joint of the index finger, all digits being bent to a considerable extent. In the Ch'en style the wrist is bent quite drastically when the hand is in a hook. Because the hook in the Wu style is derived directly from a flat hand which is pressing downwards, the wrist is bent only slightly.

In the Yang style the hook takes the form of a drooping bundle of fingertips and is also called *suspended hand*.

The Sun and the other Wu styles do not use a hook.

C. Trunk

1. Chest

Within the martial arts the chest can assume three attitudes: thrust out, concave and held. The attitude assumed in t'ai chi is held chest, or holding the chest.

The attitude of holding the chest requires that the shoulders and collarbones be relaxed, the shoulders be curled forward a little and the ribs be gathered in very slightly. The chest cavity is thus free to expand vertically and the diaphragm is able to stretch downwards as you move.

Holding the chest has no similarity with the tense retraction of a concave chest, for the feeling of a held chest is one of broadness.

The reason for holding the chest is that in t'ai chi, breathing is done from the abdomen. With abdominal breathing you breathe at your normal tempo: you don't breathe any more quickly but you breathe more strongly and more deeply so as not to run short of breath. This strong, deep, paced breathing is quite the reverse of that adopted in activities where breathing is done from the chest and the chest is thrust out.

The attitude of holding the chest does not alter as the body moves, but is fixed and stable. Since the chest is neither concave nor convex, but upright, it then becomes very easy to breathe deeply and with the diaphragm. The abdominal region and the liver are massaged rhythmically as the diaphragm thus expands and contracts, and this massage helps the blood circulation as well as assisting the liver to function more efficiently.

Holding the chest is the hoarding or reservoir attitude of the chest and performs a major role in martial arts attack. That role is to help transmit striking or dynamic power through the hands. The rotating from side to side and up and down of the chest muscles is what allows this role to be fulfilled.

Being able to guide the hands with the body and guide the body with the hands as the movements of the body revolve and rotate comes with long and thoughtful practice of t'ai chi, as does being able to have the chest rotate along with the hands. When this happens, the muscles of the chest will not only stretch out and contract but will also arc around both vertically and to each side of the body.

Holding the chest is not an easy concept to put into practice, so don't despair if it feels awkward at first. So long as you consciously avoid thrusting the chest out and work slowly towards a feeling of holding the chest a little when in a posture, you will gradually feel more and more at ease with the attitude of a held chest. If you find it too difficult to assume this attitude with the chest, however, you should be very careful that you don't develop instead a hollow-chested, hunch-backed stance.

The collarbones should be stabilised quite deliberately so as to enhance the attitude of *shielding the vitals*. This is the technique whereby, as the muscles of the chest relax down and pull around to the front, the ribs also relax down one by one. The upper half of the body is thus upright rather than loose, the body's centre of gravity is fixed and the body is quite under control.

Concrete/hollow in the chest controls the hands: this is what is meant by the phrase *the upper is closely tied to the hands*. With the chest held in slightly and the collarbones relaxed down, the muscles on either side of the chest follow an arc-shaped path, alternating between concrete and hollow as the body moves. This makes the chest much more effective from the point of view of attack and defence as well as in its transformations between concrete and hollow. And as your movements increase in delicacy and precision, the greater will be the benefit your body derives from t'ai chi.

To ensure that the leg in the hollow position will have agility, yet in no way lose its anchorage, there should be an echoing between the hollow leg and the held chest, which brings about a symmetry between upper and lower.

2. Back

According to the Chinese theory of main and collateral channels*, the *tu* acupuncture points function as overseers to other acupuncture points which have a direct connection with specific organs or parts of the body. These *tu* points are all located along the spine, starting with the *ch'ang ch'iang* point (at the base of the spine) and ending with the *ta chui* point (at the rear of the base of the neck). Also along the spine are all the *shu* points, which are the control points for the body's vital energy (*ch'i*) and blood, and which act as juncture points for the *ch'i* of the visceral organs.

T'ai chi's stress on exercising the spine promotes a balance of *yin* and *yang*, distributes *ch'i* and blood more harmoniously and removes blockages. Exercising the spine as t'ai chi does is also exceptionally good for the digestive, respiratory and metabolic systems.

Drawing the back is allied with holding the chest, and the ability to hold the chest carries with it the ability to draw the back.

To draw the back, the back muscles relax down while the

*Note: Main and collateral channels are a network of passages through which *ch'i* circulates and along which acupuncture points are distributed. Main channels are vertically distributed trunk lines, and collaterals are the large and small branches shooting off the main channels. The viscera, the surface of the body, the head and the limbs are linked into one integrated whole by the 12 main channels, 15 collaterals and 8 extraordinary channels.

chest is held in slightly; at the same time the vertebrae in the shoulder region feel as though they are lifting both upwards and very slightly backwards. It is important that they lift upwards as well as reaching backwards, and this is particularly so with the third vertebra down from the top of the back.

While the purpose of holding the chest is to enable power to be modulated at will, the purpose of drawing the back is to enable power to be both furled and released. In attack and defence they fulfil the complementary functions of releasing and hoarding.

Bending the trunk forward and backward exercises the nerves running along the spinal cord, and it is the vertebrae of the upper back (the thoracic vertebrae) which control the bending of the trunk. The primary function of drawing the back is to restrict the degree of movement of the trunk so that it does not bend more than 30° from the vertical. Its second function is to stretch the mobile muscles across the top of the back even further than during ordinary t'ai chi movements.

A strong, pliant spine lends support and control as the body's centre of gravity is being shifted. It brings a precision to postures and movements and keeps the trunk erect.

It also works in conjunction with the small of the back in two ways. One is to initiate the movements of each of the limbs so that, once in motion, there is no part of the body that is static. The other is to do with the technique of releasing power: with the spine and the small of the back acting as the mechanism for initiating movement, inner power starts from the heels, traverses the spine and becomes manifest in the fingers. Hence the descriptions *strength derives from the spine*, and *the small of the back is the prime mover*.

3. Abdomen

For the abdomen to be tranquil and for *ch'i* to sink to the *tan t'ien* (the area about 8 cm below the navel), breathing must be abdominal. Tranquility is fundamental to the practice of t'ai chi, but the reason why tranquility is important specifically to the abdomen is that if attention is paid only to *ch'i* sinking to the *tan t'ien*, the end result will very probably be an abdomen that is excessively concrete. Tranquility of the abdomen balances this condition out.

The methods of abdominal breathing are:

(a) flow breathing, where the lower abdomen retracts on

exhalation and pushes out on inhalation, and
(b) counter-flow breathing, where the lower abdomen pushes out on exhalation and retracts on inhalation.

Ch'i sinks to the *tan t'ien* when the abdomen is pushed out. Thus *ch'i* sinking to the *tan t'ien* is not an absolute. *Ch'i* alternately sinks to and rises from the *tan t'ien* as you inhale and exhale. Whether the flow or the counter-flow style of breathing is adopted is optional.

If your purpose in doing t'ai chi is to correct a specific illness, then just breathe naturally and concern yourself primarily with whether movements and postures are correct. No harm whatsoever can come from allowing breathing to be natural.

But if you are seeking to eventually coordinate breathing with movements and derive the maximum benefit from your practice of t'ai chi then you should adopt either flow or counter-flow breathing.

Abdominal breathing helps to lubricate the intestines and increases the pliability and elasticity of the muscles of the abdominal wall. With long-continued practice in alternately tensing and relaxing (being careful, however, that in the tension there is yet tranquility), the abdomen gradually becomes compact without becoming swollen, and as pliant and elastic as an inflated football in that it is able to withstand blows from the outside.

The main point to watch when starting to learn t'ai chi is to relax the abdominal muscles. Then, as you become more familiar with the movements, start to visualise *ch'i* sinking to the *tan t'ien*.

Through the arc-shaped movements up, down and from side to side of the abdomen and its alternate tensing and relaxing, the *tan t'ien* acts in the prevention and cure of diseases of the colon and of diarrhoea. It is also responsible for the prevention and cure of constipation, seminal emission, too-frequent urination and piles. The strengthening effect it has on the kidney region renders it extremely effective in the prevention and cure of diseases of the kidney.

The major factor in *ch'i* sinking to the *tan t'ien* is the movement of the diaphragm muscles as you breathe from the abdomen. It is extremely important, however, that outward form in the postures be harmonious. To achieve in full measure *ch'i* sinking to the *tan t'ien* requires that the tailbone be at dead centre, the chest be held and the back be drawn; that the shoulders be heavy and the elbows hang down; that the crown be suspended and the crotch be suspended; that the chest muscles be relaxed down in an arc shape and that each of the ribs be relaxed down and have a suggestion of pulling around to the front.

If *ch'i* sinks to the *tan t'ien* the whole time you are doing t'ai chi, eventually your stomach will enlarge. Apart from being an encumbrance to your movements as you get older, this will make you short of breath. To obviate this, alternately tense and relax the abdomen as you exhale and inhale.

When you are releasing power, *ch'i* sinking to the *tan t'ien* stabilises your centre of gravity, allows you to put more strength into the feet and adds stability to the body as it twists around and down. It enables you to use better the reactive force of the ground as an ally and make your strength more explosive, so that power is released heavily and tranquilly.

As *ch'i* sinks to the *tan t'ien*, consciously send power right through to the heels for a fleeting instant; however, you must never squat down into postures, for that brings about flaws, concave and convex shapes and disjointedness in both form and movements. Once there is disjointedness, power separates into two strands. And unless there is one single strand of power, the spirit cannot soar nor can the whole be strung together in one piece.

The key to the entire body's being able to hoard is relaxed and upright vertebrae. You will never be able to hoard and then to release if you squat down into postures and become disjointed. It is when changing from hoarding to release that particular attention must be paid to this.

4. The Small of the Back

The T'ai Chi Classic says: *The source of life and consciousness lies in the crevices in the small of the back.* The crevices in the small of the back are the kidneys, and are also called the eyes of the small of the back. Traditionally, the kidneys were believed to be the source of the body's internal vapours, hence the belief that *ch'i emanates from the kidneys.* The T'ai Chi Classic lays stress on *deeply involving the consciousness in the region of the small of the back,* the implication being that if the kidneys are strong there will be a fulness of spirit, an abundance of *ch'i*, the nerves will be clear and the eyes sparkling.

The small of the back is that part of the back at the waist and is the pivot between the upper and the lower halves of the body.

When there is a change in motion throughout the body, the small of the back is crucial in regulating the stability of the body's centre of gravity and in driving strength and power to every extremity of the body.

What is required of the small of the back in t'ai chi is that it be relaxed, heavy and upright.

It needs to be relaxed yet heavy in order that ch'i can sink right down to the *tan t'ien* and not float away from the upper torso, and so that the lower limbs will be firm and strong yet agile.

It needs to be upright so that it won't arch forward in a swayback or stick out behind in a hump. It is not the student, incidentally, but the teacher who is thought by t'ai chi adepts to have been slack when a student exhibits such serious flaws as a lowered head and an arched back. Inclining either forwards or backwards is also a flaw in the small of the back, as is inclining to either side.

Inner power can become a lively force supporting you all round rather than just on one side only if the axis of the body is neither twisted nor rickety. And the axis of the body's turning will not be twisted or rickety if the crown of the head has a suggestion of reaching upwards, thereby pulling the small of the back upright.

With the entire body relaxed, the weight of the torso is very heavy and all of it rests on the small of the back. This means that to be really strong and for the back to straighten up, the small of the back must be vertical, just as it should be when a heavy weight is being lifted up off the ground.

The small of the back and the hips should sink slightly downwards in every stance to help stabilise the centre of gravity. By means of the centrifugal force created by the revolving of the axis of the small of the back, this slight sinking down also drives inner power right through to the tips of all four limbs. Unless the small of the back is relaxed down and upright, the buttocks tend to stick out, making it impossible for the tailbone to be at dead centre. This will adversely affect the spirit piercing through to the crown of the head and strength emanating from the spine.

From the beginning pay primary attention to relaxing the small of the back and ensuring it is upright and heavy. A relaxed small of the back which is also upright and heavy prevents rigid pressing down and stiff pulling up, both of which affect the agility of the turning movements of the small of the back.

With the bow step in one of the Wu styles the torso does, in fact, tilt forward but the back and the body are still kept erect, allowing the power of the crown of the head to penetrate directly through to the heels. By thus forming a single straight line, the vertical abides in the slanting.

All of the martial arts pay particular attention to utilising the strength of the small of the back, for when this is properly utilised there is an increase in the strength which can be produced and in the speed with which it is produced. As well as this, the strength of the whole body can be concentrated in the one spot.

The small of the back is vitally important in attack and defence, but masters of t'ai chi also say: *hands, wrists, elbows and shoulders; upper back, small of the back, hips, knees, feet: nine nodes of power, each node coming forth from the small of the back.* Since the practice of t'ai chi begins with slowness and gentleness, it is very effective as therapy, especially in the treatment of diseases of the kidney, so long as the student adjusts the pace and tempo of the movements to suit his or her own abilities.

Because such importance is attributed to the trunk in t'ai chi, concrete and hollow originate in the small of the back, moving from there to the chest. As the body moves, the kidneys alternate between concrete and hollow and the kidneys govern the legs: whichever kidney is hollow, the leg on that side of the body is hollow, and whichever kidney is concrete, that leg is concrete. In other words the legs follow along below.

The principle still holds, however, that there is hollow in the midst of concrete and concrete in the midst of hollow. If there were not, then the concrete would sink too heavily and the hollow, lacking consciousness, would waft away.

In a posture, the small of the back settles downwards, which means that the power of the small of the back descends. This helps *ch'i* to sink and power to travel through to the tips of the fingers and the toes, as well as making the legs much firmer.

5. Buttocks

The physiology of the buttocks is such that they protrude slightly. If they protrude too much while doing t'ai chi, however, the small of the back will be twisted and the head will drop. Therefore t'ai chi masters talk of *restraining the buttocks* in order to make their students aware that they should not stick the buttocks up but should gather them in. This gives the natural pulled-inwards position achieved when the small of the back is heavy and upright and the tailbone is at dead centre.

The principal function of restrained buttocks is, in conjuction with *ch'i* sinking to the *tan t'ien* and suspended crotch, to make the abdominal region compact and the movement of the diaphragm in breathing more effective. Besides making the abdominal muscles more pliant and elastic, this attitude rhythmically exercises the abdomen, the intestines, the urinary system and the kidneys.

Secondly, restraining the buttocks makes it easier to keep them centred. When they protrude there is a tendency for them to skew, which removes the tailbone from dead centre.

The core of the chest and the abdomen should always be in a direct straight line with the tailbone at the very base of the spinal column as shown in **photo A** below.

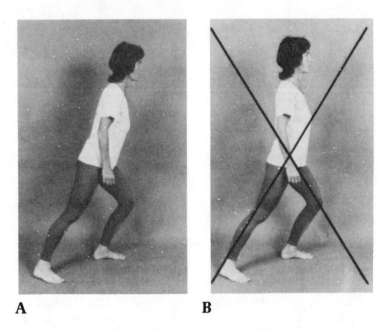

A   **B**

The tailbone acts as a pedestal on which the abdomen rests so that in whichever direction the abdomen turns the tailbone also turns, and whatever angle the movements bring the body to, an upright trunk is maintained. This is tailbone at dead centre.

Restraining the buttocks, which means tucking under the tailbone and letting it sink down, brings the body's centre of gravity down lower, fixes the lower extremity of the spine and becomes a support for the whole torso. Having this support of the tailbone at dead centre fixes the lumbar region, which adds to the spine's agility and the elasticity of the upper back muscles. This in turn enables strength to emanate from the spine.

If the buttocks are not restrained and the tailbone is not centred, but poking out, power will come through only one hand and arm. Such power will not be balanced nor will it be concentrated in a specific direction, because it is not unified power controlled by the back and emanating from the legs.

D. Lower Limbs

1. Crotch

The crotch, or perineum, is the area between the anus and the vulva or scrotum and is where the *hui yin* acupuncture point is located. The Chinese theory of main and collateral channels holds that both the *jen* (worker) and the *tu* (supervisory) pulses originate in the *hui yin* point. Therefore, the *pai hui* point of suspended crown echoing to the *hui yin* point is a natural way to open the flow of *ch'i* along these *jen* and *tu* channels.

The crotch should be rounded; it should also be hollow and not pinched tightly together. *Suspended crotch, modulated crotch* and *rounded crotch* are different names for the same thing. Since relaxed roundedness is regarded in t'ai chi as primary, it would seem best to use the term *rounded crotch* here.

If the hips are held open and the knees have a sense of being directed slightly inwards, the crotch will have a natural round-edness. But even if the knees do point slightly out, it is still possible to have a rounded crotch if the muscles along the outside of the thighs pull inwards and the hips are held open. The crotch lifting very delicately upwards with a sense of suspension in the skin of that region will render the crotch naturally hollow.

The ligaments around the hip bones are extremely strong and taut, so it is necessary to work at holding the hips really open in order that their reaching out, withdrawing and revolving will be more agile and there will be a greater scope to their movements. A hollow, rounded crotch allows the hips to be held open and is also the means by which the legs are able to make transform-ations between concrete and hollow.

The movements of the legs and of the arms are of a part: when the hands and arms go with the flow, so do the legs, and when the hands and arms go counter to the flow, so do the legs. Unless the knees are bent and the crotch is rounded, it is impossible for power to lift the heels, come forth in the legs, rise to the spine and take shape in the fingers in a continuous, regulated flow.

With the small of the back and the hips relaxed down and the buttocks slightly restrained, the crotch will be filled with easy power. When this power moves down to the feet the knees are strengthened and the tread made more stable, since the soles of the feet grip the ground more evenly and solidly. The power of the crotch descending echoes ch'i sinking to the tan t'ien, thereby making the abdomen more compact and the centre of gravity more assured.

A crotch which is hollow, i.e. hollow in the midst of concrete, lends to all revolving movements a very agile appearance. Once the power of the crotch has descended, and suspended crown has guided upwards, the body is held in the naturally upright and steady position which t'ai chi masters have traditionally linked together as the techniques of lifted crown and suspended crotch.

When power is released while the body is in motion, whether this be latent power or manifest power, there must be a transformation in the region of the small of the back and the crotch. Without this transformation it is impossible to release power correctly and with relaxed heaviness and to focus power precisely. It also helps to make faster the seeking of the straight amidst the curved in the direct shooting out of power. This transformation in the small of the back and the crotch can also regulate both the stability and adjustment of the centre of gravity, and the agility and coordination of changes in body, hands and gait.

When the trunk is lowered down, the power of the crotch rising from the tailbone is facilitated by holding the hips open to broaden the crotch and keep it rounded. But in lowering the trunk down, the crotch must at no time descend beyond the kneecaps; otherwise the strength of movements will be impaired. Because of the looseness thus created, the power of the crotch cannot be gathered in, the legs stick out uselessly and the transformations between concrete and hollow become fuzzy.

The transformations between concrete and hollow of the small of the back must be closely coordinated with open/closed and concrete/hollow in the crotch. In changing from one movement to another, the small of the back and the crotch should be easy and lively, otherwise movements will lose their nimbleness and become wooden.

Before inner power can sink down completely when either latent power or manifest power is being released, the crotch must be secured and the small of the back entwined.

If the small of the back and the crotch are neither easy nor lively, inner power will be plainly slow; if the small of the back is not sunken and the crotch is not secured, the power released will be obviously superficial and lacking in strength.

2. Hips

Of the three major joints of the upper limbs—the shoulders, the elbows and the wrists—seek first to relax out the shoulder joints. Of the three major joints of the lower limbs—the hips, the knees and the ankles—seek first to relax out the hip joints. Relaxing out the hip joints allows the action of the small of the back and the movements of the legs to become more agile and coordinated.

The aperture between the pubis symphysis and the joint on the sciatic node* is expanded when the crotch is rounded and the hips are relaxed out. By thus enlarging the scope of movement, the arc-shaped movements of the legs are enlivened and inner power is able to rise up into the small of the back and the spine. It is by these means that a certain degree of opening out of the hips is achieved.

If the hips are opened out too much, however, or if the hips descend to knee level when the torso sits back, the aberration known as swaying crotch will be produced. The primary effect of opening the hips out too much is a slackening in the tensile strength of the body whereby the legs have no solid foundation and stretching and withdrawing strength lose their bite.

If the hips are not opened out enough, the aberration known as pointed crotch will be produced: this prevents lively advance and retreat.

The hip bones are the crucial points in regulating movements of the small of the back and the legs, and it is extremely important to relax the hips open.

Since the hip is where the small of the back and the leg actually meet, insufficient relaxing open of the hip bones, which leads to woodenness, makes it very difficult for the small of the back and the legs to move in concert. The small of the back is the

---

*Note: Pubis symphysis is the midline joint between the two pubic bones, and the sciatic node is the hip and thigh joint.

axis of the body's very delicate turning movements and, because of its close proximity and structure, the pelvis must also turn very delicately with the small of the back. In other words, to turn the small of the back is in fact to turn the small of the back and the hips together.

Because that part of the body around the hips supports the weight of the upper body, more time should be spent on exercises which loosen the hip joints than on those which loosen the shoulder joints. Such basic exercises as leg kicks, bending forward from the waist, stretching the legs (by attempting to do the splits, then turning the torso around to press down with the hands on the knees and where the thigh meets the groin) and lifting each knee in turn and clasping it to the chest all help to loosen the hip joints and increase agility and flexibility.

For the more adventurous and already comparatively fit students who want to push themselves a little further, the following niceties of gait can be worked on.

As you are about to step out with one leg from a posture, the hip of the solid foot turns along with the small of the back, rotates inwards a little and sinks down as the posture is lowered, imperceptibly. Do not allow this to destroy the single thread of upper and lower, though.

At the same time, the other leg slowly reaches out, the posture being raised the tiniest fraction as that leg reaches the midpoint of its travel. When the foot reaches and touches the ground, the centre of gravity gradually transfers on to it and when the actual posture is achieved, the hips and the small of the back sink down.

This is a very effective means of increasing the amount of effort expended in practising the modern, uniformly slow t'ai chi. It is a way of moving which gives exceptional stability to the gait at each and every point and is a technique which secures the lower part of the trunk as though it were a great tree held steady by its deep roots.

The analogy of the body as a great tree with trunk soaring up and roots boring down is completed when, with upper and lower on a single cord, suspended crown reaching delicately up and the power of the small of the back and the crotch sinking down, inner power penetrates to the very soles of the feet. Those who practise t'ai chi for a very long time using this technique develop strong thigh muscles and legs. It demands expertise and great effort, however, and should only be attemped by the really fit or by those who are seeking to increase their strength.

In order to maintain the sense of upper and lower on a single cord in all movements, the hips should be upright whether the body is advancing or retreating. They advance in unison, retreat in unison and initiate change evenly. They operate precisely in harmony with the shoulders at all times. All of this ensures that the tailbone is kept at dead centre throughout.

The movements of the Ch'en style of t'ai chi are overtly powerful. It is when learning the Ch'en style that students are encouraged to isolate individual postures through which the release of power can be practised and transformations in the small of the back and the crotch can be perfected. The purpose of this is to gain training in how to release power correctly, especially as it relates to the small of the back and the crotch.

Precision in the movements is sought first, and the focusing, speed and increase of explosive strength is the next goal. The sequence in this training, then, is to practise power before practising skill, and to practise flow before practising power. In order to increase its quality of rotation and penetration, the releasing of strength must be as rapid as a whirlwind. Only when this is achieved can skill be pursued, for *unskilled boxing is vain.* Practising with a partner is also very useful when you are experimenting in releasing strength.

The other styles of t'ai chi have now done away with movements where power is released overtly. This has been done so as to render t'ai chi suitable for use in recuperation and is the major alteration made to adapt it to widespread use.

However, there are several isolated postures which can be selected out by those who wish to train themselves in releasing power. Examples of such postures which require the coordination of the small of the back and the crotch and are suitable for training in the release of power are:

Grasping the Peacock's Tail: this movement calls for taut power, stroking power, pressing power and pushing power;

Stroking the Wild Horse's Mane: this movement calls for pulling power, splitting power and leaning power;

Unrolling the Body Punch: this movement calls for a punch that flows with the tread and advances;

Moving Block Punch: this movement calls for a punch that bends with the tread and advances.

Many of the postures in t'ai chi which are executed on one side only may also be isolated out and practised on both sides. For example, *Grasping the Peacock's Tail* could be done first in the right hand style and then carried onto the left hand style, making the two into a symmetrical movement to give the body more balanced exercise.

The vast majority of movements in t'ai chi are executed slowly, the only fast style being the Cannon Punch Ch'en style. But when postures are practised in isolation for training in releasing power, they can be performed at speed. The ability to move both slowly and quickly which is thus developed is what is meant by the injunction in the T'ai Chi Classic: *in a crisis respond with rapidity, otherwise move slowly.*

While the hip of the concrete foot is pulling very slightly inwards and sinking down and the hollow foot is slowly extending outwards, there should be both a differentiation between concrete and hollow and a split second when the hips are held fully open.

If, with the shifts in motion in each and every posture, the small of the back is lively and the hips are open and if, in completing each and every posture, the small of the back sinks down and the hips subside, the hips will eventually begin to relax open of themselves. When this happens, the turning movements of the small of the back and the legs become exceptionally nimble and the tread becomes much lighter and expanded.

3. Knees

The legs carry the weight of the whole body while it is in motion, but it is the knees which bear the greatest burden of this weight. The knees, therefore, must be strong yet nimble.

In t'ai chi each foot acts in turn as the support for the body's centre of gravity as steps are taken. When the hips turn and are held open, the knee moves along with the foot which is stepping out as it lifts up, slowly steps out and turns. So the burden on the knees is much greater than in those martial arts in which movements are made quickly. Agility of movement is also heightened by the continual gyrations of the hip and knee joints.

For the beginning student, pressure on the knees is lessened by the adoption of a fairly upright stance in which the knees are bent only a little.

When stepping out, first raise the thigh—not the foot itself or the whole leg—of the hollow foot so that the strength thus concentrated in the knee acts to raise the heel.

When doing a kick or a one-legged posture, first raise the leg, concentrating strength in the knee. The kneecap should be lifted at least to hip level, and as the ligaments of the hips stretch it can gradually be lifted to as high as the heart. A good loosening up exercise is to stand on one leg and hug the other knee to the chest with both hands. By thus stretching and loosening the muscles you will gradually find it easier to bring the knee up higher in one-legged postures and to make kicks higher and freer.

Concentrating strength in the kneecap when raising the knee allows the strength and power of the entire body to permeate right through to the tips of the toes, greatly adding to the releasing of strength. The releasing of strength can be vastly increased when the hips are held open, the muscles alternately contract and stretch and the joints are soft yet pliable.

The arc-shaped transformations of the legs between concrete and hollow are flow encirclings and counter-flow encirclings which are guided by the gyrations of the hip and knee joints. The legs and arms act in concert in weaving an encircling web. Do not misinterpret this as simply a matter of bowing or bending a straight thread, however. It is this encircling web which is the crucial factor in the complete integration of the whole, from foot to leg to spine to its taking shape in the fingers, as well as being the source of the nimbleness and pliability of the hip and knee joints.

In relation to the knee in the art of attack, the T'ai Chi Classic comments: *when (another's) foot approaches, (I) raise (my) knee*, and *when in close, use the knee*. *When (another's) foot approaches, (I) raise (my) knee* means using your own leg to sabotage an opponent's leg. It is a protection for the crotch and the shinbone and a counter to another's raised leg, as well as being a way in which the knee and the leg can be used for both attack and defence. *When in close, use the knee* means that in kneeling stances or stances where the knee is hurled inwards or outwards, the kneecap is lifted in order to attack with the knee and to bring an opponent to the ground.

In a posture, there should be a sense of the knees hooking very slightly inwards. In front and behind, or to the right and the left, the knees respond to each other and, in coordination with the open roundedness of the hips, focus the power of the crotch. This is the closed residing in the open and, as well as protecting the crotch, it brings to the lower part of the body a heavy strength.

When the foot in front has trodden firmly on to the ground the kneecap must be no further forward than the toes of that foot, otherwise your equilibrium will be upset. Nor should the kneecap and the shinbone form a vertical straight line, for that affects the liveliness of the movement that follows. What the knee should do when the front foot is bowed out is extend a little further forward than the vertical but not at such an angle as to protrude out past the toes.

4. Feet

The feet are the foundation on which is built the style and technique of taking steps. If the foundation is unstable and incorrect, then the style and technique of gait will be messy.

There are simple steps, complex steps, large steps and small steps in the various styles of t'ai chi, but they all without exception call for precise, lively and stable movements of the feet. Discipline in the style and technique of taking steps supports and adjusts the stability of the body's centre of gravity. It also obviates ungainliness and enhances easy breathing.

Where the hands advance three parts, the feet advance seven; Victory lies in advancing and holding your position while not being vanquished lies in retreating and avoiding the full force of an attack. The point of these aphorisms is that the way the feet are used is of primary importance.

Advancing: The heel of the foot that is stepping forward lifts off the ground first. The toes hang down as that foot is moving, then curl up slightly to allow the heel to be placed on the ground first. Once the heel has made contact, the sole of the foot treads down and lastly the toes.

Retreating: When stepping backwards, the heel of that foot lifts off the ground first. The toes of the retreating foot, however, touch the ground first, followed in turn by the sole of the foot and then the heel.

Half-step: Where the rear foot moves forward towards but not past the front foot, the heel of that foot lifts off the ground first. But either the toes or the sole of that foot are placed on the ground first and then the heel.

Stepping sideways: The heel of that foot stepping sideways, e.g. in *Cloud Hands,* is lifted off the ground first. When that foot is placed down, the toes touch the ground first, followed in turn by the sole of the foot and then the heel.

When about to step out with either leg, the small of the back and the abdomen first incline around in the direction that leg is going to take, and the groin pulls in slightly towards the back.

Weight is supported wholly on the one bent leg, the strength of which is in the front thigh muscle. The buttocks are directly above the heel of the supporting leg and the strength in the buttocks transfers down to the heel to increase the firmness of the knee in that concrete leg without sacrificing its flexibility. The stance is thus extremely stable and firm.

The trunk is lowered very slightly, then the other leg gradually stretches out without quite straightening the knee. The strength of this hollow leg is also in the front thigh muscle. With the toe consciously guiding the path of the foot, the body rises imperceptibly when that foot is halfway along its path so as to add to the strength of the movement and avoid rigidity.

The heel of the leg which is stepping out is placed on the ground first. The stride should be light, moving slowly across with the weight of the body as the whole foot treads down.

The feet take the weight of the body in turn so as to maintain the body's equilibrium.

The toes, the sole of the foot and the heel all tread evenly on the ground, with the point just behind the ball of the foot kept high, when the ankles and legs are rotating. In this way the concrete foot presses down heavily as if rooted to the ground and gives firmness to the stance while the hollow leg is able to change agilely.

When you are about to step out to the left, the right kidney sinks down as the right hip draws in, thus allowing the left leg to step much more lightly. The same applies in reverse when you are about to step out to the right. This is a practical example of the second of the Five Principles of Symmetry and Accord, that *intending to go to the left, you must first go to the right; intending to go to the right, you must first go to the left.*

In the original Ch'en and one of the Wu styles, all turning movements involving the legs adhered rigidly to this pattern. As t'ai chi has developed in recent years, however, many turning movements involving the legs do not necessarily conform to this pattern. The other Wu style currently practised has in fact dispensed with the leg describing an arc as a step is taken. The reason for this is to make t'ai chi easier to learn and to make it more suitable for the older and the frail.

Although the feet move alternately, there should never be a complete cessation of movement. All movements should be arc-shaped, possessing at all times a spiral strength; as the hands revolve, so the feet flow along with them, moving in a spiral.

Hence the saying, *the feet go along with the motion of the hands.*

Cloud Hands as it is practised in the Ch'en style illustrates this principle very clearly.

In *Cloud Hands* the left foot takes a wide step to the left, describing an arc as it is lifted up and placed down. When the body's weight and centre of gravity have transferred across on to the left foot, the right foot describes a similar arc as it, too, takes a wide step to the left. However, just as it is about to be placed down alongside the left foot, the right foot is retracted a fraction towards the right before actually touching down on to the ground.

In other words, the movements with the feet are arc-shaped, not straight. This applies to each and every movement with the feet in t'ai chi.

The coordination in *Cloud Hands* between upper and lower in getting power moving in a spiral through the hands and feet is as follows:

As the left foot steps out, the left hand travels up from the right rib cage. It then circles across to the left in front of the face. The palm is facing in and obliquely up and the path followed by the hand should be no higher than the top of the head.

As the hand moves, inner power twines obliquely out from the armpit along to the hand, moving from the thumb through each of the fingers in turn until it reaches the little finger. It will then have completely filled the hand.

The movement of the left hand to this point is described as flow turning. The turning point between flow turning and counter turning is that instant when the left hand reaches the furthest point of its leftward travel and the palm turns face down.

During the second half of the circle travelled by the left hand, down (no lower than the hips) and along across to the right groin, inner power twines obliquely back into the armpit. This part of the movement is counter turning.

With the right hand, inner power twines out from the armpit down into the hand as the right hand pulls up from the groin and passes to the right across the face (flow turning) and twines back as it arcs down from the right shoulder and then to the left across the lower body (counter turning).

In the legs, inner power twines down out from the hip to the toes as the left foot moves across to the left: this is flow turning. The twining back in and up to the hip of inner power while the left foot remains on the ground is counter turning.

With the right leg it is the same: inner power twines out and down to the right foot as it arcs across to the left (flow turning) and twines back while the right foot remains on the ground (counter turning). Flow and counter turning is reflected in the knees as they turn outwards away from the crotch (flow turning) and inwards towards the crotch (counter turning).

Cloud Hands is one of the postures extracted by practitioners of the Ch'en style as an isolated posture in which to train themselves in releasing power. If this movement is performed rapidly it becomes a ball of snapping strength with both hands moving in circles and the body weaving from left to right. In attack and defence it has the dual function of toppling an opponent by ensnaring his or her front foot and of striking sideways with both hands.

The original purpose of the legs moving in an arc in the martial arts was to ensnare legs, entrap feet, kick knees and shinbones, tread on feet, alight on weak spots, etc. It was also used to prevent an opponent using those tricks and making a further attack.

The characteristic t'ai chi movements of reaching out in an arc or in a circle with the legs, turning the toes up, down and to the right and the left, are all extremely beneficial to the joints of the feet. These actions also open the flow of the main and collateral channels and increase pliability and agility in the joints of the legs.

The lifting up, placing down and turning to the right and left of the heel is woven inextricably into the fabric of the whole cycle of movements, as are the turning up, pointing down and hooking in and out of the toes. These rounded, smooth movements have been developed not only to look graceful but also to develop a nimbleness in the joints of the heel that can both prevent and alleviate flat feet, a point of special importance to middle-aged and older people.

The power in the big toes guides all the up, down, in, out, forward and backward movements of the toes. The direction in which the toes point plays an important part during turning movements in determining the extent to which the hips are held open and how much energy is expended. For this reason it is worth studying each posture individually to make sure that the toes of the front foot are pointing directly ahead of the body and not out to the left or the right.

Take, for example, *Grasping the Peacock's Tail—Right* as it is executed in the Yang style. If, as the right foot lifts up and is about to move forward, the toes of that foot point to the left or left front rather than straight ahead, the opening out of the hips will be affected such that the hips will be crimped in tightly, while the whole body will incline a little to the left rather than bearing straight ahead when the posture is achieved.

The direction in which the toes point is quite important and attention should be paid to their turning and their direction at point of contact with the ground in every posture.

You should become very aware of the interrelationship between limbs and trunk and how each affects the other, realising that inattention to minute points can impair the precision of the overall movement of the body. If the toes of the leading foot point in any direction other than straight ahead of the body, it will be impossible to have *three tips in relation.*

With the movements of the upper limbs, the hands guide the elbows and the elbows guide the arms. With the lower limbs, the feet guide the knees and the knees guide the thighs. The crucial factor is that the fingertips and the tips of the toes very delicately guide the motion of the hands and the feet; if stiffness intrudes, nimbleness will suffer.

The chest and the abdomen should go along with the movements of the feet and hands as well, upper and lower accompanying each other as one integrated whole. When the toes point directly ahead, the hands should also point directly ahead, just as the gaze should be towards the front. This is another aspect of upper and lower accompanying each other, the aim being to line up upper/lower/left/right in the one direction and centre the entire body into a strong entity.

Attention should also be paid to stability in advancing, retreating and turning, and abrupt changes in body height assiduously avoided. Greater expenditure of energy is thus made possible and paces will be kept to a uniform size and the correct angle of steps retained.

E. Joints

During all movement in t'ai chi, consciousness should be directed towards relaxing the joints, stretching the ligaments and increasing flexibility and agility. This conscious relaxing and stretching ensures that movements flow consistently and smoothly into each other.

At the same time, the technique of bringing the joints into proper alignment with each other allows them to work more smoothly and firmly as well as distributing body weight more evenly over the skeleton and increasing strength and stamina.

A word about relaxing and contracting as it operates in t'ai chi. Relaxing is a natural letting go which becomes softness; contracting is a natural changing from the relaxed state into one of tension, which then becomes hardness. The movements of t'ai chi are such that the joints continually alternate between a state of relaxing (always somewhat longer) and a state of tension (always of shorter duration).

The basic point to keep in mind from the start is to relax out the hip and shoulder joints so that the joints of the arms and legs will move more freely.

With the spine, it is very important to relax out the upper back and the small of the back. The small of the back—because that is where the *ming men* acupuncture point, which also bears the name the *gate of vitality* and which is regarded as the body's centre, is located. The upper back—because attached to this part of the spine are the ribs, which should sink down and pull around to the front so as to enhance *ch'i* sinking to the *tan t'ien*.

Gradually, as the whole body relaxes, every joint in the body should also be relaxed out. This relaxing out of every joint can become a reality in t'ai chi because, with the small of the back initiating them, all of the complex revolving, stretching and withdrawing movements of the limbs flow on to stretch the entire body: *in moving, there is no place that does not move.*

It is particularly important when a posture is struck that the joints be properly aligned in order to give the body greater support. Relaxing of all the joints should go hand in hand with their very delicate alignment so that a sense of free, open movement is retained. The vertebrae and the major joints have to be relaxed out before the body can flow powerfully and agilely. Fundamental to t'ai chi is the concept that the body is a whole made up of its parts, a family: *vitality springs from a reunited body.*

The joints of the limbs should be curved and holding a little in reserve rather than being straight, rigid or stiff: *by means of the curved, power and to spare is stored*, and *relaxing out my power, I cannot then be subdued.* The capacity to be completely still when you are still and to be movement incarnate when you are in motion presupposes that curve which stores power and to spare.

This, in conjunction with the transformation of inner power having the closed residing in the open and the open residing in the closed, is a prerequisite for the skill of being instantly able to move quite freely and with strength when taken by surprise. The ability of t'ai chi masters of old to retaliate instantly and accurately no matter from which direction an attack came was the result of their developing this hoarding or storing attitude.

The power of the entire body climaxes simultaneously in the instant of reaching each completed posture. All the joints come to rest in a symmetry of right with left and with a harmony between upper and lower. The hands, feet, etc. come to rest in symmetry; the hands and the feet, the elbows and the knees, the shoulders and the hips, the breasts and the sides of the abdomen all harmonise with each other, the open is completely open and the closed completely closed.

The ceaseless turning, alternating between open and closed and concrete and hollow, which a complete cycle of t'ai chi entails, allows the muscles and ligaments to subject the joints to the ideal amount of alternate relaxing and tensing.

Appendix

88-Posture T'ai Chi Cycle

Section 1
1. Preparatory Stance
2. Rising
3. Grasping the Peacock's Tail—Right
4. Single Whip
5. Raised Hands
6. Crane's Wings
7. Brushing the Knee Twist—Left
8. Strumming the Lute
9. Brushing the Knee Twist—Left, Right, Left
10. Strumming the Lute
11. Advancing Block Punch
12. As Though Sealing Up
13. Crossed Hands

Section 2
14. Embrace Tiger, Return to the Mountain
15. Oblique Grasping the Peacock's Tail—Right
16. Tip of Elbow Punch
17. Reverse Unfolding the Arms—Left, Right, Left
18. Sideways Flying
19. Raised Hands
20. Crane's Wings
21. Brushing the Knee Twist—Left
22. Needle Pointing to the Bottom of the Sea
23. Ducking through Arms
24. Revolving Punch
25. Advancing Block Punch
26. Step Up to Grasp the Peacock's Tail—Right
27. Single Whip
28. Cloud Hands
29. Single Whip
30. Testing the Horse
31. Separating the Feet—Right

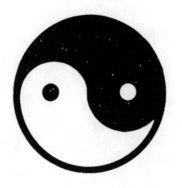